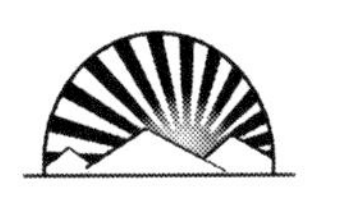

TESTIMONIES

"What you get in this book from Morris Keller is that most uncommon of all qualities in the modern world: common sense. It is the basis of all healing modalities which are not married to machinery, poisoning, cutting, or burning away the symptoms of illness. And Morris' common sense is married to spiritual practice, whatever your religion. There is much in this book which is useful to the person seeking to do as the Scriptures suggest: Physician, heal thyself."

—Red Hawk
Poet, Author, English Professor, U of A, Monticello
Self Observation: The Awakening of Conscience

"When knowledge, wisdom and experience come together in a book, it is a treasure and a great service to humanity. Dr. Keller's book is full of practical and timeless teaching understandable to all."

—Dr. Rosita Arvigo, DN
Author, International Lecturer and
Director of Ix Chel Tropical Research Center, San Ignacio, Belize.

"Wow, what an eye-opener to understand our health from this perspective. Everyone should realize the impact our environment and diet have on our health. The holistic approach Dr. Morris Keller reveals in this book will enlighten even those, as myself, who never think much about health. My attitude and understanding of the whole realm of being healthy has changed now. This book is a must-read for everyone willing to face the truth about their health."

—Pastor Richard Deeds,
Fountain of Life Church, Belize

Fountain of Life Church
Vision Statement

Our mission is to reach the lost and equip the found. Our passion for ministry is to bring emotional healing to hurting people and to restore broken and wounded relationships. Our compassion is to those whose lives lack identity, purpose and destiny, to lead them to the true "fountain of life", Jesus Christ.

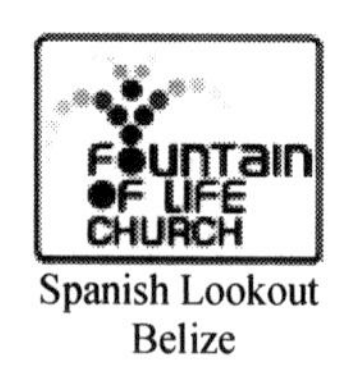

Spanish Lookout
Belize

As members of the Fountain of Life Church, Dr. Morris F. Keller and his wife, Kathryn Rose, are committed to the above statement and their desire to bring healing to others by helping to bring several interconnected factors into balance. Each of us suffers, to a greater or lesser degree, either from a chemical, nutritional, physical, emotional or spiritual imbalance—each of which affects each other thus producing stress and illness. We can achieve balance by making lifestyle changes and by partnering with God.

Monies earned both by the publisher and authors from the sale of this book will be used to fulfill this health ministry.

Setting Yourself APART from the

SEEDS of CANCER

A NATURAL HEALTH and SURVIVAL GUIDE

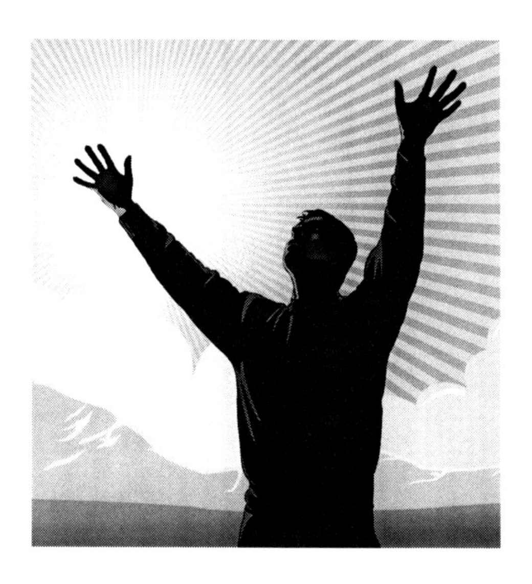

Dr. Morris F. Keller
Kathryn Rose Mandel-Keller

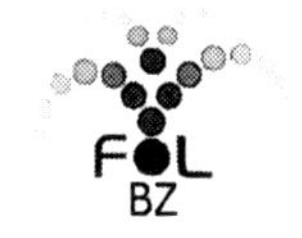

Fountain of Life Church
Spanish Lookout, Belize

Copyright © 2010 by Dr. Morris F. Keller

All rights reserved, including the right to reproduce this work in any form whatsoever, without permission in writing from the publisher, except for brief passages in connection with a review.

First Paperback Edition May 2010
Revised July 2010

Published by the Fountain of Life Church
Box 198
Spanish Lookout, Belize C.A.
E-mail: folchurch@fountainoflifebelize.com
www.fountainoflifebelize.com

Distributed by
Ingram Book Company
One Ingram Blvd.
La Vergne , TN USA 37086

Cover art © by Gino Santa Maria
Cover design by Kathryn Rose Mandel-Keller

www.naturalcleansingtechniques.com

ISBN: 978-976-95291-1-3

Printed on acid-free paper in the
United States of America

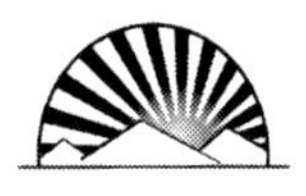

DEDICATION

Both Rose and I would like to dedicate this book to my Father, Myron, and to my Grandfather, Joseph, whose deaths from cancer had set me on this path of wellness. Had it not been for their fate, I might not have chosen a natural healing for myself, nor would I be in a position to pass this knowledge onto others with the hope and faith in God that they too can be healed.

So, for the love of Jesus, we also dedicate this book to Him and to all those seeking to eliminate the seeds of illness in their lives as well as restore or discover their own personal connection with God.

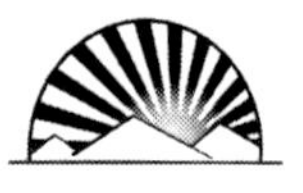

NOTICE

The teaching, instruction, claims, recommendations, suggestions, information and products mentioned in this book, via email, conversation and/or through associated web site pages, have not been evaluated by the United States Food and Drug Administration and are not approved to diagnose, treat, cure or prevent disease. The information provided in this book, via email, conversation and/or through associated web site pages is for informational purposes only and is not intended as a substitute for advice from your physician or other healthcare professional. You should not use any of this information contained in any latter forms of communication for diagnosis or treatment of any health problem or for prescription of any medication or other treatment. You should always consult with a licensed healthcare professional before starting any diet, exercise or supplementation program, taking any medication, or if you have or suspect you might have a health problem.

Quoted Bible verses are from:

The King James Version Reference Bible

Unless otherwise stated

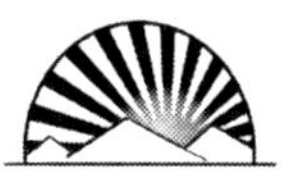

TABLE OF CONTENTS

Appendices

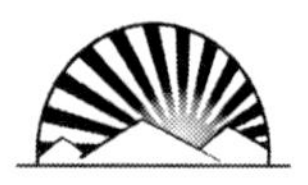

ACKNOWLEDGEMENTS

I had heard many times over the years that writing a book was ten percent inspiration and ninety percent perspiration. This book would never have happened without my wife Rose. She has been the ninety percent which includes research, writing, editing, layout, artwork, indexing and marketing—to name most of the "hats" she has worn. I am not as computer savvy and I could not have accomplished this project without her by my side. During this process, we have learned much from others and from each other that has strengthened our marriage.

We have been most blessed to have benefited from our readers whose input all caused correction or change in our manuscript. Thank you: Dr. Robert "Red hawk" Moore, Dr. Rosita Arvigo, Matthew Miller and Pastor Richard Deeds whose perception and attention to detail is greatly appreciated.

Many thanks go out to all of our students over the years who have shown us and others their commitment to natural healing, shared their results and have encouraged us with the evidence that these less-often utilized methods—along with lots of practical advice—continue to work and provide much hope to others.

—Morris F. Keller

I especially want to thank my husband, Morry, for teaching me what I know about natural healing, supporting a healthy lifestyle, for putting his trust and faith in me and my ability to coach others and to contribute fully to this book. Thanks also for your fabulous cooking while I stayed busy at the computer and for not complaining when other things were left undone. I'm grateful that we work as a team.

Additional thanks goes to Jeanny Plett and her assistance with PhotoShop and the inside header design, Alisha Deeds for the FOL logo, Mervin Budram and Glenn of TAS Belize for their tremendous patience and effort to transfer my cover design to templates in InDesign until I was satisfied, and our friend, Pastor Ed Kurtz for taking the back cover photo of us on March 27, 2010 at Alisha and Randy's wedding—a very blessed event.

Special thanks to Susan Brill of The Winsome Word for authoring our news release to the Christian market, for editing our hard cover and revised soft cover edition, and for taking a personal interest in our story.

All illustrations were obtained from dreamstime.com. The following list credits each individual artist:

I.......... Blood Cell: © Kandasamy M. p. 29
II......... Skeleton: © Betacom-sp p. 32
III........Muscles: © Linda Bucklin p. 34
IV........Circulation: © Danny Photo 80 p. 35
V.........Lymphatic System: © Sebastian Kaulitzk p. 37
VI........Nervous System: © Oguzaral p. 39
VI-a.....Skin and Fat: © Oguzaral p. 40
VI-b.....Lungs: © Talisalex p. 42
VI-c.....Digestive System: © Andreus p. 44
VI-d.....Endocrine System: © Oguzaral p. 46

I also want to thank all the folks in Spanish Lookout—who are too numerous to mention—who have come to know us and accept us and have been an inspiration to us in writing this book.

—Kathryn Rose Mandel-Keller

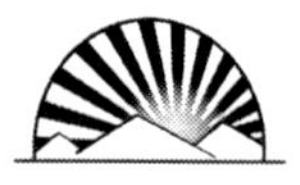

"But know that the Lord has set apart him that is godly for himself." Ps 4:3

Preface

Our message is to provide proven, practical answers for what may sound foreboding to some and yet realistic and to be expected to countless others. There is a critical need for change however; there is no need to actually fear. Our Lord says (Is 41:10):

> *Fear thou not; for I am with thee: be not dismayed; for I am thy God:*
> *I will strengthen thee; yea, I will help thee; yea, I will uphold thee with the right hand of my righteousness.*

Knowing that our Lord will look out for us if we trust in Him, we must now look at some facts. Our planet is in crisis. The combination of floods, droughts, fires, earthquakes, volcanoes, melting polar ice, rising seas, rising temperatures and man's inhumanity to his fellow man, coupled with new and ever changing strains of viruses and bacteria, is a convincing argument that our planet is in crisis.

Most of us are familiar with this definition of "cancer": a malignant tumor that tends to invade surrounding tissue and spread to new body sites. But are you aware that the American Heritage Dictionary also defines it as, "a pernicious spreading evil"—pernicious meaning deadly or destructive. We all have the seeds of cancer but not all of us will develop the disease of cancer. However, the odds are greatly increasing due to the self-destructive nature of humanity—we are the only animal that spoils its own nest with garbage and pollution. The seeds of cancer exist all around us and they are being allowed to germinate and spread in our thoughts, in our bodies, in our actions and in our societies unless we decide to change. Will you be shielded from the influences and the effects of a cancerous world?

There is a prophecy that only one third of us will survive, according to Zechariah 13:8–9. Now, many of you may be thinking that this verse refers only to the inhabitants of Jerusalem and what is now the land of Israel. However, as we read to the end of Zechariah, we discover that all nations will suffer great losses. When? We don't exactly know. But you do not have to be a Bible scholar or a scientist to perceive that something is terribly wrong at this time. If you want to survive, be healthy and be in service to God, you immediately have to begin setting yourself apart from the rest.

This is a good place for me to interject my thoughts on what is meant by "service to God". Service to others ***is*** serving God. Everything we do and are asked to do is an opportunity to give our best according to our own God-given abilities. It is our choice and responsibility to use these gifts not just for ourselves but for the benefit of others. The true meaning of "service" is to do something at our own expense—not just when it is most comfortable, convenient or mutually beneficial. So, the next time you are called upon to serve in some way and you do not feel up to the task, pay attention to your thoughts and feelings and decide instead if it isn't more important to joyfully submit and praise God for the opportunity to discover what He has in store for you.

In order to help you to be "up for the task", our mission is to teach you the necessary health and survival techniques for this twenty-first century, not just from concepts, but by way of our personal experience and what we have already taught to hundreds of others. To accomplish this goal of health and survival, you must be confident that you can "go it alone" with God as your partner. You must relinquish the need to belong, fit in or be one of the crowd. Perhaps you may even need to leave behind friends and family in order to be true to yourself and more importantly, in service to God.

Is the effort required by my previous statements worth it to you? To be a part of a new and glorious Kingdom of God here on earth, to change others by changing yourself, and to bring along our youth to take our place, is this worth the effort to you? Or, are you just too comfortable with your present lifestyle and beliefs to change? Perhaps you are feeling that your salvation is assured and so why bother to prolong your life? Personally, I feel just like many other Christians do, as well as some non-Christians, that our God has a plan for each of us. We need to look for, discover and fulfill this plan before literally "throwing in the towel" by allowing the health of our body to deteriorate. God uses each of us to fulfill His larger plan and no matter how small of a role we have, it is a significant one. We are all held captive by this world one way or another. Paul says, "For the weapons of our warfare are not carnal, but mighty through God to the pulling down of strongholds..." (2 Cor. 10:4) Can you begin to let go and let God, undo formed opinions and lifestyles, and allow yourself to be non-conformed to the world?

This book challenges you to set yourself apart.

Dear reader, I feel compelled to tell you, straight from the start, what this book is not. If you are looking for quick fixes and sound byte answers, this guidebook is not for you. We are not marketing what might hope to be the latest fad. There is no product or anything discussed in this guidebook in which we have a financial interest. My wife and I are not seeking to enhance our own lifestyle. We feel richly blessed with the simple comforts that God has provided us. We sell nothing, except this book and our personal counseling with the proceeds mostly going back into fostering our mission and serving our Lord.

I am old enough to remember what it was like before there was TV. Our small family of three would engage in more conversation. We would read more books. We would gather around the radio and listen to news, major sporting events and mystery stories. It seems to me, the pace of life before television was slower, more patient and relaxed. TV changed our attention span capability. When the television set was on, no one could focus on anything else. The next innovation that came along, the remote control, made even more of an impact on our society. We now had the ability to quickly switch from one program to another and not even leave our chair. Advertisers and television program producers began to realize this and created quick, attention getting visuals to keep you from zapping your remote.

This only escalated with the advent of the computer, the internet and the mouse. We now have more power to click rapidly from anywhere to anywhere and our attention spans have become even shorter and shorter. We have become a "bottom line society", wanting quick answers in short form. We flit from one enticement to another, never willing to delve deeply into anything that takes time and patience. In order to become self-sufficient at anything, however, you must develop patience and perseverance. This is particularly true of natural healing which works gradually—not instantly. My prayer, for all our readers, is that you will continue to delve into the contents of this book and glean the following from it:

You will…

Learn how to prevent and heal yourself of Cancer and other illnesses in partnership with God.

Learn how to attack the cause and not just the symptom of disease

Learn how your body works.

Learn the simple causes of Cancer and most illness.

Learn simple self-help proven methods to address and reverse disease.

Learn how diet and lifestyle changes can create healing.

Learn how to create delicious healthy meals.

Learn how to free yourself from drug and medical costs.

Learn how pre-natal and post-natal nutrition determine wellness.

Learn how to rejuvenate your body and increase longevity.

Learn how to make health a daily, personal responsibility.

Learn how to reduce stress and increase stamina.

Learn how to re-balance yourself chemically, nutritionally, physically, emotionally and spiritually.

Learn how to downsize your lifestyle and become more self-sufficient.

Learn to appreciate God's wisdom and the truths of the Bible.

This book will also provide you with my insights gained from personal experience in financial security, growing your own food and making better choices affecting your health and survival.

The rewards or payoff from this investment in your education may very well be your key to survival as our current civilization is now in turmoil. "And it shall come to pass, that in all the land, saith the Lord, two parts therein shall be cut off and die: but the third shall be left therein." (Zech 13:8) This book is not a message of "gloom and doom". This Natural Health and Survival Guide is a message about a better tomorrow and how we can help pave the way for Christ's New Kingdom on Earth. It is the product of many years of personal research and knowledge gained from hundreds of students and the divine inspiration from Father God, whom I seek to serve.

This is not a book of scientific discourse designed to meet the research criteria of academia. It is more about my revelation than my education. I sincerely pray that the ideas put forth herein will speak to your heart as being truth.

The forgotten lesson taught to all new medical students is, "First of all, do no harm". In my opinion, the lessons and methods taught in this guidebook should always be employed before any radical therapy is considered, since the methods herein will do no harm.

The chapters of this guidebook will lead you on a systematic path to develop your confidence and skill in personal health management and the lifestyle changes necessary for your survival. Prevention of illness and maintaining wellness is what we seek, which is better than waiting until a health crisis forces us to make radical changes.

Do not be surprised that most of what is taught in this book is not taught in conventional medical schools because self management of health is not profitable for doctors, hospitals or drug companies.

Our intent is to awaken your overall comprehension of how your body works and what it takes to keep it running as it was designed by God. My own path has taken me on many quests. It seems to me that the more I learned, the less I knew. Medical schools teach a very narrow focus of illness and health. Some have finally conceded that lifestyle may be a factor, but what lifestyle? Our work, pleasurable activities, diet, environment, relationships, even our thoughts and spiritual health all play a significant role. Much has already been spoken of and written about lifestyle change and its effects on health. It comes at us from all directions with the advent of modern technology and mass media. We are a people, community, nation and world in search of answers. But, are we just being fed what “they” think we want to hear? How can we possibly get at the truth?

I have been a seeker of truth all of my life and I have finally come to the conclusion that we have already been given all of the answers we need through the Word of God. Man does not have to reinvent and reprocess what has already been created in nature in order to find a cure for whatever ails him in life. We just need to get ourselves out of the way (stop interfering and messing things up) and let God's unique design resume control and simply assist by following His ever-wise instructions. The Bible should be our first source for answers.

As we read our Bibles, we discover that our bodies are designed to last 120 years or more but to achieve that takes careful maintenance. The ancient Israelites, such as Moses and Abraham, lived well beyond our average lifespan of today. Have you ever asked yourselves why that is?"

One explanation is more scientific than the other. Our planet has undergone many changes since ancient times. The air, water and soil were cleaner then. The spin of the earth on its axis may have been truer then. Now, because of the "wobble" that has been created by underground nuclear test explosions and dams that hold millions of gallons of water, our globe is spinning off center. This is like the armature of an electric motor being out of balance. The frequency or vibratory rate of our planet has changed.

I also believe it is because the Jews of the Old Testament obeyed the laws and covenants of God—at least some did most of the time, all did some of the time but none did all of the time. Despite their sinful nature, God's dietary and hygienic instruction prevented disease and prolonged their health and well being. Adam and Eve, Abraham, Moses, and Jesus were all fit and healthy. The Jews never got the illnesses of their Egyptian masters because they set themselves apart. There were no fat prophets or disciples, as far as we know—they are not depicted. Today, these Words of God are mostly ignored and believed to be overridden by the coming of Jesus and the Lord's Grace and His gift of salvation.

To the contrary, Paul wrote to the Romans (Romans 7:12), “Wherefore the law is holy, and the commandments holy, and just, and good.” Jesus did not come to do away with God’s law but rather to do away with the religious ritual and sacrifice. His was the ultimate sacrifice. Our salvation is assured once we accept Jesus as our Lord and Savior. However, our health in this body is not so assured.

At this point, I would like to just begin to touch upon a subject which we will call “Divine Healing”. It is my belief that God can end or prolong your life in the body at any moment, if He so chooses. The phenomenon of “faith healing” has always reinforced the omnipotence of the Lord for me, whenever I have personally seen it happen. We all need to walk with God every moment and our first reaction to any situation needs to be to pray. If God chooses not to give you instant healing then perhaps He needs to see some effort on your part. We will have more to say on “Divine Healing” in Chapter Three.

Our ability to serve our Father in earnest is handicapped if we do not honor the body He gave us. God gave us a user’s manual for His creation, namely the Bible. Leaving no stone unturned, He has instructed us on the proper maintenance of our physical, mental, emotional and spiritual well-being for optimum performance. When we are negligent and disobedient and follow our own choices and worldly desires, it may not affect our salvation but there are consequences both in this life and I believe in the life thereafter—I believe that we are rewarded accordingly.

Perhaps, with closer scrutiny of how our body works, we can develop greater understanding of how awesome our God is and how precious is the “Temple of the Holy Spirit” and know what we can do to preserve it and use it in praise of Him, Christ Jesus.

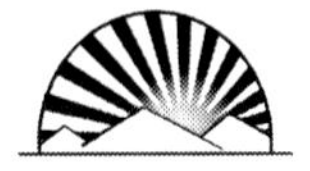

Introduction
My Victory Over Cancer

There are no accidents—something has led you to pick up this book. Likewise, something has led me and my wife to make it available for you to read. Each new day's experiences are built upon the preceding day's experiences and so life becomes a sum of many experiences, lessons learned and discoveries along the way. In this respect, our lives are similar and yet we both know that each of us travels a unique path. Where does it lead and what is the point of this individual journey? These are two big questions most of us seek to answer, myself included. We tend to look everywhere but at the obvious. Sometimes we avoid it like the plague. "Religion" becomes a touchy subject. For me, however, I looked in many directions in order to find truth and purpose in my life. Finally, after absorbing the ups and downs and ins and outs of what life has to offer, you begin to piece things together that start to make some sense and it brings peace and satisfaction to what might have been a rough ride. You find from the many studies, encounters and personal insights that there really is a meaningful reason for all this to take place. I found my answers by paying closer attention to what I felt the Lord was trying to tell me.

My story and spiritual journey have led me to become a health missionary in God's service. We each need to discover a purpose for living rather than just existing. When we greet each day with joy we are taking the first step on the path to better health. This philosophy, purpose and mission in your own life will set you *apart* from most of humanity.

How I started out on this journey called "life"…

As we are nearing completion of this book, I am approaching my seventy-second birthday—born October 6, 1937 in Providence, Rhode Island. My mother later told me how significant and difficult my birth was to her since she had lost another boy prematurely before me and one again after me. I now believe that God was setting me apart from birth. Only one third of my mother's children survived. There is no logical reason why I should be alive now except that God wants me to serve Him.

At any time in my seventy two years, God could have snuffed out my spark of life. There are many instances from infancy to now, when serious accidents and illnesses could have easily ended my physical existence. From a very difficult birth, falling down flights of stairs as an infant, bicycle crashes, boat capsizes, teen age drinking, physical risk taking, cancer, drug experimentation, falling off a cliff and even more recently, when Rose and I first moved to Belize, we were hit by an oncoming vehicle at high speed and survived without a scratch on us. Our vehicle did not fare nearly as well. I think by now, you should get the idea that perhaps God has a better plan for me.

My parents were Jews of European heritage. As an only child, I received more attention (mostly disciplinary) but was expected to "be seen and not heard"—an attitude which probably came from the Elizabethan era in England. Consequently, I spent much of my time alone—either in my crib or playpen as an infant or in my bedroom or fenced-in back-yard as an adolescent—left to my own amusement. Perhaps God set me apart even back then.

Babies gurgle and coo and cuddle their teddy bears and I was no different. However, from infancy, I remember talking to a "friend" both out loud and in my heart. It is my belief that babies perceive more than adults and those special abilities have been programmed out of them by society. Vaguely, I remember seeing an "angelic" shape by my crib. When I tried to tell my mother about my "friend", she cautioned me not to tell this to others because they might think I was "crazy". Nonetheless, I continued to seek the love and companionship I felt while communicating with this presence I perceived came from God. Today when I meditate on God, I set myself apart in order to better perceive what my Lord is trying to tell me.

You may find the following statement controversial: I believe that Divinity resides in us from conception and that the "conscience" or Holy Spirit that tried to guide my life then and now is our Lord Jesus; after all, we are made in His image. David said, "For thou hast possessed my reins; thou hast covered me in my mother's womb." (Ps 139:13) Did I have the innate desire and will power to always say and do the righteous thing? Of course not! In human flesh, we are naturally born to sin. Only as we mature and finally come to realize that Jesus paid dearly for all of our sins and when we can accept Him as our true Messiah and Savior, only then, are we aided with the inner strength and guidance of the Holy Spirit.

To be born a Jew is quite another matter entirely. I was never taught to seek a direct personal relationship with God. Instead, I was taught that The Messiah was not Jesus and, most assuredly, that the Jews were God's "chosen people". Chosen for what, I always wanted to know?

From ancient times, Jews usually lived near and socialized with other Jews, mostly relatives or members of the same temple or synagogue. My generation lived the same way. They set themselves apart and except for school time friends and business customers, our family never associated with gentiles. Their lifestyle, however, appeared to be no different than the people they set themselves apart from. What you did for a living and how much wealth you acquired seemed to me what interested my family most. My role models drank whiskey and smoked cigarettes. My father was a middle income physician/foot surgeon and I was expected to join him in his private practice when I grew up. A prospect I thought safe but uninspiring.

We did all the things expected of a middle class Jewish family. We went to temple on the two high holy days of Rosh Hashanah and Yom Kippur. We sat in our reserved seats in the more prestigious original building and it seemed to me as a child that most adults were more interested in what their counterparts were wearing in the way of furs and expensive clothes than they were in being thankful and repentant. Occasionally, we went to Temple on Friday nights to celebrate the Sabbath. Singing the old Hebrew hymns was the best part for me since I love to sing. Our religion seemed to be one of heritage and obligation rather than one of inspiration and communion. My wife, Rose, shared the same experience as a Jew and I wonder how many others did too?

What is the truth? The very first thought that comes to the mind of most Christians is that of Jesus who said, "I am the way, the truth, and the life: no man cometh unto the Father, but by me." John 14:6. Additionally, we find in John 8:31–32:

Then said Jesus to those Jews which believed on him, "If ye continue in my word, then are ye my disciples indeed; And ye shall know the truth, and the truth shall make you free.

What a blessing it is to come to know Christ Jesus. We can absolutely trust in His Word since His very nature is truth and He can not tell a lie. Man, on the other hand, is very prone to lies. Lying has become more commonplace than most of us realize. It has infected all parts of our lives. You know, it is one thing to tell an outright lie, but people try to skirt around it in so many ways—with little white lies; giving false or misleading impressions, insincere promises or any other means of the bending of the truth. In this way we are constantly being manipulated or manipulating others. Who is profiting? We need to re-evaluate our own motives and the motives of others so as not to succumb to the coercions of this world. A good standard to use in determining the truth in this world is to follow the money trail.

Personally, I have come to the realization that truth is the final answer to the question, Why? From earliest childhood, I experienced confusion when adults did not like to answer the question, Why? I perceived that adults did not like to answer, "Why?" because they would have to reveal the truth when they were living a lie—most adults were living double standards. They would say one thing and yet do another. Adults were and still are uncomfortable when a child asks, "why?" Sadly, this appears to be even truer today due to the harried and busier lifestyle and perhaps, even more so, due to the absence of a God driven consciousness where we take the time to teach good principles to our children. This indifference on the part of my parents also seemed to be the same with teachers and friends. Early school days held little interest for me because of my questioning, rebellious nature. Friendships seemed very superficial and life was filled with uncertainty except for the comfort I always found with my heart felt friend. What a friend we have in Jesus.

Death impacts my life's direction …

My first experience of a death in the family definitely set other things in motion for me. While I was in high school, my paternal grandfather died at age seventy-six of colon/pancreatic cancer after several years of various surgeries terminating in a bag he wore outside of his abdomen. My grandfather naturally relied on the practices of western medicine since he had medical training in Russia before he came to the U.S. as a refugee. Since his status in a new country did not permit him to practice medicine, he began selling life and health insurance while retaining his mindset that one will undoubtedly come to depend on the services of the medical establishment and eventually die.

This same role model, either directly or indirectly, changed the course of my life. As a young boy in elementary school, my recollection of my grandfather was as a sick man unable to work much. And yet, he attended synagogue regularly. It was his strong Jewish faith that kept our family bonded to our religion. While he was yet alive, I could not openly deviate from my Jewish heritage which included Hebrew training for Bar-Mitzvah at age thirteen. I suspect that the death of my grandfather released my father from some self imposed Jewish obligation because shortly thereafter, my father sent me to a Quaker prep school and then to a Catholic college for pre-med training. Probably, this was as much for disciplinary reasons as anything since I was still a very rebellious person.

My explanation of why my father directed my education in this way is this: When my father first opened his medical office in Providence, he hired a young lady who came from an Italian family and neighborhood to be his assistant. Consequently, instead of a practice of mostly Jewish patients, as was the norm for Jewish doctors, my father treated mostly Catholic, Italian people. Perhaps one of his patients encouraged him to change my educational path but whatever the real reason was, it was never confided to me. As a result of this shift, I received my first serious exposure to Christian friends and the Gospel of Jesus Christ. A wall of separation from gentiles came down.

Singing has always been a love of mine from childhood. I sang my bar-mitzvah service at temple with organ accompaniment, a role usually performed by the cantor of the temple. However, my favorite songs seemed to be Christmas carols sung at school each year. Choir, glee club and choral singing also became a part of my extra-curricular activities in high school and college. Whenever there was some religious event at Quaker prep school or Catholic college, the choir was always called on to perform. At each institution, there were congregational baptisms using the sprinkling of “holy water”. I gave my life to Christ during these ceremonies, and during communion but it certainly did not have the same meaning to me as it does today despite the fact that the Bishop came from Boston with holy water from the Pope and performed a special baptism.

From my Jewish perspective, back then, it seemed liberating to be a Christian. One could not only eat all the forbidden foods like bacon, ham, sausage, shrimp, and lobster, but one could also be forgiven of any wrong doing by asking God for forgiveness and accepting Jesus as the

Messiah and one's personal Savior. How comforting, I thought, though shallow compared to the understanding I have now. I still had much to learn. First there must be a death of the old self and a re-birth in Christ.

A Fork in the Road…

In 1957, during my second year in Podiatry School at Temple University in Philadelphia, my father, like my grandfather, was diagnosed and operated on for colon/pancreatic cancer. This was a life-changing period for me.

We had access to many of the best medical experts who consulted on my father's illness. Specialists from noted clinics and hospitals came to confer. It was a mind blowing experience, as a lowly sophomore medical student, to listen intently to these "gods of medicine" discuss my father's illness and for me to come to the shocking realization that they did not know any more about how to heal my father than the "man in the moon"—nor do they know any more today despite many years of research and billions of our dollars spent.

I began my own research program when my father died six months later. I read every book in the medical library that I thought might contain some clue as to why my father and grandfather had died of the same illness. I found no answers there.

It was the year 1959 when my high school girlfriend became my fiancée and we soon married. Together, we decided that I should drop out of medical school and go into the Army to fulfill a compulsory obligation at that time. I continued to read a slew of books on health and religion since reading was always my passion. In 1961, after my wife graduated from college we decided to move to Cleveland, Ohio to resume my medical training at Ohio College of Podiatry. I worked nights and went to school days while my wife held a position as a daytime juvenile probation officer until she became pregnant with our only child, a son. Eventually, we moved to Dallas, Texas after my training, where I began a private practice in my specialty of Podiatry/ Foot Surgery.

All during this time my inner voice still counseled me but I had sort of become a free spirit and paid it little attention. I wasn't making much time for God. Life then was mostly about financial survival for me, keeping up payments on a large bank loan, satisfying an ego to be a highly respected foot surgeon, and maintaining a lifestyle that included membership in an exclusive Jewish country club. Once again this left little time for wife, family or God.

Crisis brings change ...

Three years later, in 1969, I was diagnosed with what appeared to be an ascending colon tumor with probable invasion into adjacent organs and glands like the liver and perhaps pancreas, a hernia in my diaphragm and other "suspicious looking areas". Since x-ray—following a barium "cocktail"—was the first diagnostic tool employed, exploratory surgery to confirm the diagnosis was advised, but my inner voice said, "***no***". I was already convinced that I was in serious trouble.

I knew immediately that I was not going to go the route of my father and grandfather who had died from this same cancer. And, I also knew that I needed to do an "about face" in my life. I had no idea what I was going to do, but I needed to change. Unfortunately, this mindset caused me to ask for a separation—and later a divorce—from my wife until I knew what I was going to do and how I was going to support myself, her and my six-year-old son as well. My practice suffered from neglect, I took a bankruptcy, and then sold my practice to an associate in order to be free of financial obligations. The stress of maintaining a costly lifestyle had been removed, but my health problem had not been really addressed. I had neglected my spiritual health and much more.

As I reflect on this period of my life it is with mixed emotional feelings of guilt and remorse for violating the sacredness of my marriage and not being a proper father to my son. For this I have asked forgiveness and repented.

I began going to church singles meetings soon after my divorce and began dating a divorced lady (whom I later married) with an eight-year-old son. She gave me a paperback book by Adele Davis about food and nutrition. This first step in the direction of natural health spoke to me and convinced me that there was an important link between diet and health. I began to make changes in my dietary habits and became more selective in food choices, but intuitively knew that there was so much for me to learn, it seemed almost hopeless.

I began praying for guidance by asking my inner voice for help. I guess I totally surrendered to a Higher Power for the first time in my life. Just days later, an issue of the "Guardian" newspaper had an article about a dentist who had healed himself of colon/pancreatic cancer with natural methods and was teaching others. Praise the Lord! What seemed even more remarkable was that this dentist was now living in Grapevine, Texas, just sixty miles from me. I praised the Lord again!

Dr. William Donald Kelley had a small dental office located in his home on a quiet street in Grapevine, but Dentistry was only a front for his cancer research. He was a student of Beard (a British researcher) in the use of pancreatic enzymes for cancer and analyzing various blood markers to track progression or regression of cancer cells. He developed a dietary questionnaire that could be analyzed with a computer program and published a manual that told his patients what to eat and how to begin to cleanse and detoxify their bodies. This included coffee enemas, to which I was at first repulsed. At the time, I questioned his rational for this procedure but never received a satisfying answer. Not until much later did I learn that he had gotten this protocol from Dr. Max Gerson. Having long overcome my earlier attitude, I have to this day made an enema a part of my early morning regimen because I have come to value the numerous benefits and the refreshing start that it gives me each day.

Some of you may be shocked and find this hard to believe. I guess after almost forty years of daily enemas, it never occurs to me as strange—especially, after teaching it to many, many others to preserve their health. It may interest you to know that a number of years ago a very well-known cancer specialist from Sloan Kettering Cancer Center in New York, Nicholas Gonzalez MD—a name some of you may be more familiar with—did a research project with the same Dr. Kelley who had taught me. Gonzalez published his findings in the most respected medical journals after several years of integrating Kelley's protocols with those of the establishment. He found great improvement in the groups he integrated. For those of you still doubting me, Gonzalez also wrote that he himself had derived great benefit from the program and had incorporated the daily coffee enema into his morning routine.

Within six months on Kelley's program, I began to feel much improved, but knew I was barely "half-way home". Over the next two to three years I investigated and applied the teachings of Drs. Max Gerson, Bernard Jenson, and Carey Reams to my personal regimens and began to develop my own personal program that incorporated the best of all the above with some personal modifications—constantly refining and updating. Our synergistic/holistic program that we offer to our students today combines the essence of proven protocols developed by Drs. William Donald Kelley, Max Gerson, Bernard Jensen and Carey Reams. Here is an account of my personal journey to discovery...

Dr. William Donald Kelley.....

In 1969 (the same year I was diagnosed with cancer), Kelley had published his own book, *One Answer to Cancer*, after going through his own personal battle with pancreatic cancer. In it, he presented a dietary program taken from his own experience and further research. It soon became a best-seller in the "nutritional underground" and antagonized those in "orthodox medicine". While opposing my own medical background, I concur with Dr. Kelley, that the root cause of cancer is the body's inability to metabolize (digest and utilize) protein and a lack of minerals. Of course, I did not know it at that time but having gleaned it as well from my own healing experience and further investigation, I support the belief that proper protein digestion plays a critical role in eliminating and preventing further cancers. In William Kelly's own words:

> The person gets cancer because he's not properly metabolizing the protein in his diet. Then, to make matters worse, the tumor has such a high metabolism that it uses up much of the food which is eaten. If a

> person's disordered protein metabolism is not corrected it will give rise to more tumors in the future, even if the first one is successfully removed. This, by the way, is the unfortunate reason why so many seemingly successful cancer operations end up in recurrences a year or two later. The tumor was removed, but the cause—improper protein metabolism—remained.[1]

Dr. Kelley's linking of faulty metabolism to a deficiency of pancreatic enzymes that are more readily associated with digestion in the small intestines, was actually a continuation of the work of a British physician named Beard, who concluded that these same enzymes are secreted into the bloodstream where they reach all body tissues and digest cancer cells—the very cells that block our immune system from functioning. Dr. Kelley also identified mineral imbalance as a root cause of the breakdown of the immune system. These three factors: pancreatic enzymes, mineral supplementation and enema detoxification greatly influenced my own natural healing of colon/pancreatic cancer. The more I learned about God's intricate design of our bodily functions and what can cause them to break down, the more I understood the process of natural healing.

About one year later, after my introduction to the protocols of Dr. Kelley, someone who knew me gave me a book about Dr. Max Gerson. He was a German born physician who came to New York in the 1920s and was healing people of cancer with fresh vegetable juices,

---

[1] "Kelley's Nutritional-Metabolic Therapy" (c) 1993 by Richard Walters- Excerpted from Options: The Alternative Cancer Therapy Book, Avery Publishing[1]

cleansing diets and coffee enemas. In a lecture given in Escondido, CA in 1956, Dr. Gerson stated, "I am convinced that cancer does not need a "specific" treatment. Cancer is a so-called degenerative disease, and all the degenerative diseases have to be treated so that the whole body at first is detoxified."

I proceeded to add Gerson's protocols to Kelley's and felt another part of the puzzle had been found....

Dr. Max Gerson...

Much has been written about Dr. Max Gerson—a famous German physician who fled Nazi Germany to New York City in the 1930s. Gerson began his journey of discovery of natural healing, while still in Germany, by finding a dietary cure for his own severe migraine headaches. When one of his patients using his "migraine diet" discovered that it had also cured his skin tuberculosis, Dr. Gerson was encouraged to do further research with diet. He then went on to successfully treat many other patients of tuberculosis. Along with the help of Dr. Ferninand Sauerkraut, a famous thoracic surgeon, the "Gerson Treatment" became established as the first published cure for skin tuberculosis.

Dr. Gerson then attracted the friendship of Nobel Prize winner Albert Schweitzer, M.D., by curing Schweitzer's wife of lung tuberculosis after all conventional treatments had failed. Gerson and Schweitzer remained friends for life. Dr. Schweitzer followed Gerson's progress as the dietary therapy was successfully applied to heart disease, kidney failure, and finally to cancer. Later, Schweitzer's own type II diabetes was also cured by following Gerson's therapy treatment. Dr. Albert Schweitzer went on to praise Dr. Gerson when upon his death in 1959 he said, "He leaves a legacy which commands attention and which will assure him his due place. Those whom he has cured will now attest to the truth of his ideas."[2]

Basically, the Gerson Therapy is a natural treatment that boosts your body's own immune system to heal cancer, arthritis, heart disease, allergies, and many other degenerative diseases. By consuming large amounts of organic fruits and vegetables and freshly prepared juices throughout the day, the body is provided with a mega-dose of enzymes, minerals and nutrients that break down diseased tissue and rebuild healthy tissue while coffee enemas eliminate the lifelong build-up of toxins from the liver.

Well, my natural curiosity and persistent drive to find the truth of something would not allow me to stop here. I had to ask myself, "Was there more to completing this methodology of healing the body naturally?"

Dr. Bernard Jenson...

Again, several years later I came upon a book by Dr. Bernard Jenson about tissue cleansing written in conjunction with Victor Irons: *Tissue Cleansing Through Bowel Management*, 1981. After trying this technique, I achieved greater results than before and incorporated this into my own health and teaching program. From 1986 to1992, I was director of nutrition at a chelation clinic in Arkansas and we purchased so many of Bernard Jenson's books for our patients that Dr. Jenson came to see us personally and spent two days with me at the clinic. He

---

[2] Quoted from: http://www.gerson.org/about/mg.asp

gave me many of his own personal insights from years of experience that I use and treasure to this day.

Dr. Bernard Jensen began his career as a chiropractor in 1929 and then turned to the practice of nutrition in search of remedies for his own health problems—sounds familiar? Dr. Jensen believed that nutrition is the greatest single therapy to be applied in the holistic healing arts and to the whole patient—not just to the treatment of a disease. These are my exact sentiments, as well, since treating the disease or symptoms does not eliminate the cause. Wellness stems from the whole body being in balance supported by a lifestyle in balance. In all, Jensen worked with over 350,000 patients around the world. He traveled to over fifty countries to study the lifestyles of the different cultures. He wanted to understand the principles of long and healthy living. He studied the long-lived people residing in Russia. The oldest man he met in Russia was 152 years old which is reminiscent of ancient times spoken of in the Bible.

Mostly what I gained in knowledge from Dr. Jensen was the concept that disease begins in the bowel where years and years of accumulated toxins and putrefied, hardened waste matter prevent absorption of nutrients and leech poisons into the blood stream that are carried to all parts of the body seeking to do havoc where we are most susceptible. So, not only is detoxifying the liver important with coffee enemas but so is a special cleansing program that literally "cleans house" and cleanses the colon, organ and gland systems.

Dr. Carey Reams...

One of the last pieces of the healing puzzle came to me when I was introduced to the Biological Theory of Ionization in 1985. I had always suspected that pH (acid/alkaline) balance was a key to health. Dr. Reams made pH balance a cornerstone of his teaching. In my surgical training, we were taught about maintaining electrolyte balance during surgery, but never considered it thereafter. Carey Reams was a pioneer in teaching urine and saliva testing as indicators of pH balance and diet for correction thereof. He also taught how to perform simple tests for sugars, salts, albumin and nitrogen.

Dr. Reams was persecuted by the medical establishment because his mission was to empower mothers to be the health maintenance resource of the Christian family unit. What actually got him into trouble was that he had been practicing medicine outside the scope of his license which was Veterinary Medicine. As a devout Christian, he was more concerned with helping people than making money. After achieving success by applying his own research to animals, he continued to teach his ideas to his brothers and sisters in Christ who came to him as volunteers.

An overview of the lessons learned...

When cancer cells are grown in the lab, there are two things necessary for growth. The two substances are acidic and sugar medium. This is true in the body as well and many natural health researchers, including myself, believe that acidosis and toxicity causes most illness as well as a lack of minerals to provide enough electricity. This relates directly to the food we eat. Simply said, all foods are either alkaline or acidic—an over consumption of one or the other throws our body chemistry out of balance. This forces our internal systems to attempt to compensate and make adjustments that most often result in undesirable consequences.

So unless you are willing and determined to change your diet, detoxify and cleanse your body, balance your body chemistry, and moderate your lifestyle to maintain health, you will continue to suffer from environmental and lifestyle affliction of disease and illness. Genetically speaking, we each have our own individual susceptibilities to disease but we actually bring illness on ourselves.

Cancer free…

Finally, after integrating all these protocols into my own regimen I was completely healed and have remained cancer free and in very good health ever since. It has been nearly forty years since I was diagnosed with a "death sentence" and I feel that I am in better health today then I ever was despite some normal aging that I haven't discovered a cure for. However, you can definitely slow down the aging process and prolong your life and live more productively into "old" age by applying what I have learned.

Now, what would you do if you were able to heal yourself of a life threatening illness? You, like me would probably want to tell as many people who would listen to you all about it, right? That is exactly what I wanted to do. However, I was still a licensed physician and my licensing board of examiners told me that I could not hold a license and practice outside the scope of what was being done in my area or what I had been taught in school. So, what would you do then? I told my board of examiners that their license was of no use to me anymore and they told me to "be careful because you can be arrested for practicing without a license". And so, I became a teacher not a doctor. For many years I sort of "went underground" and offered to teach only carefully selected students. We had prospective students sign a form that made them attest to the fact that they were not working for any government agency and that they were taking full responsibility for their own healing.

Over thirty-five years later, I have not only healed myself but also taught hundreds of people how to heal themselves of almost every illness including cancer, diabetes, arthritis, cardiovascular disease, infertility and more.

But, the important thing is where this has led me to the present time. As my health gradually improved, my desires for unimportant things lessened. In 1983, divorced and single again after my second wife and I chose to go on different paths, I moved to the mountains of northwest Arkansas into the heart of the "Bible Belt" seeking a more healthful lifestyle than living in or near cities. I had no specific plan in mind other than to go where I felt God was leading me. A strong feeling that has always guided my life is this: if one seeks a higher path that others are not ready to follow, then sometimes family and friends have to be left behind with love and blessings. Magically, doors opened for me and I opened a mostly vegetarian, natural food restaurant in a tourist town. We won statewide recognition when featured in a newspaper. I gave free cooking classes and natural health seminars at the restaurant. I formed "Mountain View Natural Health Association", a cooperative effort among local businesses and family farms to create a small eco-tourism industry and a local mid-wife/pre-natal counseling service.

A treacherous misstep helped lead the way…

Shortly after opening the restaurant, while hiking in the mountains with a friend, I stepped out on a precipice overlooking a river valley and due to loose shale rock under my feet fell over the edge eighty feet to the rocky slope below.

The first impact came after a sixty-foot drop. I had tucked myself into a ball going over the edge and my left forearm hit first, then my forehead. The force of this first blow sent my body another twenty feet through the air. At this time, I became aware that I was watching myself from some higher place above. I was being drawn towards the brightest, most comforting light I had ever experienced. From books I had read, I realized that I was going through a near-death experience. I remember either speaking out loud or to my inner Spirit, “But I cannot die now Lord, I have too much to do in your service”.

The next thing I remember is being huddled in a heap among rocks, bushes and brambles at the bottom of the cliff. When my eyes slowly opened, I was looking down into my left forearm that had been torn open. The bone was visible as well as muscles and tendons. I dared not move anything until I could determine what else was damaged. It took my hiking companion about fifteen minutes or so to reach me. I instructed him to leave me lay still while he went for help. I was back in my body but not so sure that death would not have been a better option than what the immediate future held for me. My best guess would be that it was thirty minutes or more before help returned. During this time while I lay motionless and perhaps paralyzed at the base of that cliff, I had a re-birth as I prayed for my life and rededicated it to the Lord, Jesus Christ as my personal Savior. The tears poured down my cheeks, but I could not wipe my eyes or blow my nose. Whatever the old me was, I left it behind that day on the rocky slopes and a new me was born again, re-dedicated to a life of service.

By the time help arrived, in the form of four friends with a blanket and tarp, I had regained some sense of being alive and realized that I, with God's help had to take control of this situation. I asked not to be touched until I could determine what portions of my body were working or not. I began to attempt to move individual fingers and toes and realized that they worked and had feeling. Next, I cautiously tried to slightly move upper and lower extremities and realized that they could move but not without extreme pain and spasm in my abdomen and everywhere else.

Very slowly over the period of about an hour, with my instructions, I was able to aid being moved onto a blanket/tarp litter and carried down the remaining slope, across a creek and into the back of an SUV where I was driven to the local small hospital. There they insisted on starting an IV, sewed up my arm, packed it in ice and sent me off in an ambulance to a bigger hospital about forty-five miles away.

There must have been a sedative of some kind in the IV in addition to just saline solution, as I do not remember anything else until I awoke in a hospital bed with an x-ray machine over me taking snapshots. I overheard someone in a scrub suit saying something about "exploratory surgery" for a possible ruptured spleen and more.

I was then told, as I became more awake, that I had six "burst fractures" of the vertebra in my neck, some cracked ribs and a big hole in the front of my left shin bone near the knee. The internal damage could only be determined by "opening me up".

"Stop everything," I said. The attendants were in shock as I pulled the IV out of my arm and asked for some distilled water, some oranges, and a phone to call my friends to "get me out of here before you kill me". I knew the same God who helped heal me of cancer and who returned me to life after falling off the cliff could be counted on once again to guide me back to health.

It took about an hour for my friends to come for me. I had to sign many forms releasing the hospital from responsibility for my life. My friends drove me back to the room where I was living above the restaurant, got me some purified water, oranges and Vitamin C. I lay in pain and spasm on a mat on top of a hardwood floor for the next twenty-four hours, praying, drinking water, eating oranges, taking Vitamin C and trying to crawl to the toilet in the next room when I felt an urge, but nothing came out.

The next day, I was able to hobble down the stairs and very slowly, with the aid of a hiking staff, walk about four blocks to a local chiropractor who was trained in acupuncture. He used many needles in many places on my body and when I left there, the pain had lessened. By the time I got back to my room, I could barely make it to the toilet, having been relieved of the spasms of my kidneys, bowels and bladder which earlier prevented any release. Praise the Lord! One more acupuncture session and ten days later, I was able to hike back up to see where I had fallen. I praise the Lord again and again! I believe I had a ***miraculous*** healing! The acupuncture alone could not have enabled me to heal so quickly. There was a Heavenly Hand involved.

Reconnecting with Mom…

In 1985, my seventy-eight year old mother came to live with me after consigning her second husband, with Alzheimer's, to a nursing home. We both lived in town in a small house she had bought while I continued to operate the restaurant. We also lived part time, out in the rural countryside in an Amish community where I taught the Elder Brother to heal himself of prostate cancer. Within a few months, he was much improved. Over a two year period, we continued to spend several days at a time in their farm community where I learned the skills of small family farming—a self-sufficient lifestyle. I also attended many on-farm workshops held around the state by the organic growers association, where I began to grasp the rudiments of sustainable agriculture. At the same time, I resumed Bible study with local Christians, once again raising my awareness of the Holy Spirit within.

My mother was also a good help to me in the restaurant until we both accepted an offer to work at a chelation clinic in a nearby town. We did this for four years. During that time, in 1988, I was reading an issue of a natural lifestyle magazine, when I learned of "desem" (naturally leavened) style bread. This ancient craft of baking had been taught in Europe to several bakers who had just returned to the United States. I was intrigued and delighted to discover that one such craftsman was located several hours north of us in Salina, Kansas. I contacted him and he graciously invited us to come for a visit. This became the first of many pilgrimages as I continued to apprentice under him in order to become an artisan baker. We then opened our own artisan bread bakery—in the same neighboring town as the clinic—using a wood fired brick oven that I had hand built. Business was good. And more importantly, we were making a positive difference in the health and diet of our patrons…but more on this in a later chapter.

In 1994, we sold the bakery and our home in order to once again move further north and west to join a new community that was forming. I was seeking clean air, water and soil, the opportunity to build my own home from my own design, learn organic agriculture from a master farmer, and start a healing retreat. I am blessed to have also found my true "soul mate", Rose, by way of a personal introduction from a friend in Florida. She soon joined my mother and me in Arkansas. I am grateful that she was there during my mother's later years. The three of us enjoyed some wonderful experiences together and Rose later was most helpful in ways that would have been awkward for me. I was blessed to be able to care for her as long as I did. My mother, Minna, died at age ninety-six about two years following hip surgery and a couple of strokes.

Rose and I have been married twelve years at the writing of this book. We became immersed in agriculture and crafts—which we sold at a regional farmer's market—when our mission of teaching health and healing was not in high demand. This period, however, greatly increased my understanding of local farming and organic agriculture which you will discover as you read further along.

Arriving in Belize…

In 2003, Rose and I felt that the Lord was telling us to seek a place to relocate outside of the USA where our skills and teaching might be more appreciated and needed. We investigated Cuba, then Mexico and Guatemala before being drawn to Belize in 2005, by what I believe to be divine guidance. As a result of an idle conversation during lunch at a restaurant, a man from the Mennonite community of Spanish Lookout sought me out where I was originally preparing to build our home. He agreed to become a student and learn to heal naturally of his colon cancer. Then a relative of his, with the same cancer, came to Spanish Lookout from Canada with his family and stayed three months while I instructed him as well. As a result of the improvement in the health of these two students, in 2006 we became the only non-Mennonites (and Jews) ever invited and approved by the committee of representatives to live in the community of Spanish Lookout where we now reside. We now know that God's hand was once again behind this move for the purpose of immersing us in a culture committed to living a life by the Word. Our renewed personal acceptance of Jesus as our Lord and Savior has enabled us to see the spiritual imbalances affecting the health of our students.

Our direction now as health missionaries is to reach out wherever we can to bring our message to as many churches as possible by way of health seminars called "Taking Care of God's Temple". These seminars and the material taught in them have been the inspiration for this book. If you feel that your Church would benefit from one of our seminars, please fill out the request form on our web site: www.naturalcleansingtechniques.com/howtoheal.html. As we travel, we would be open to visiting churches in the same area.

Teaching natural healing methods and healthy lifestyle choices is my purpose and goal in life. Having rejected a grim prognosis at age thirty-two, I had made it my mission, back then, to research these methods of natural healing; to discover what factors contributed to good health; and to live the healthiest lifestyle I could. Now, forty years later, cancer-free and still thriving, my mission is to pass this knowledge on to others so that they may choose a healthy long-life over an early death-sentence, just as I did.

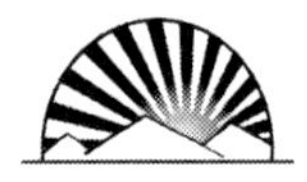

Chapter One: **How Our Body Works**

Nothing in the Universe except God Himself is more intricate in design than the human body and we are made in God's image.

I can still remember the first time I saw a holographic picture, created with a laser on glass. You could smash the glass image into hundreds or thousands of pieces and each fragment would still retain the original whole picture. It is my belief that every fragment of our body contains the whole imprint of God.

Every currently known and yet to be known engineering and scientific principle occurs in the human body. The list is almost endless including, the lever, block and tackle, fulcrum and wedge, liquid hydraulics, combustion, osmosis to name just a few.

It is not our intent to educate you in conventional anatomy, physiology, or any other medical science in this chapter. Instead, we want you to visualize the human body as a wondrous gift from God and with that gift, comes the responsibility to keep ourselves healthy.

Most people know more about their cars and other vehicles than they know about their own body. And, most people definitely take better care of their cars and trucks than they do their own body. We want our car to last as long as possible and give trouble free service.

Do we have the same desire of our body? We may have the desire but are we willing to consider that maintaining a healthy body is similar to maintaining a healthy automobile? The highest quality fuel will make a vehicle run better. Preventive maintenance will protect against untimely breakdowns. These same principles hold true for our body as well as our vehicles up to a point.

An automobile mechanic said to one of his customers who also was his personal physician, "Why is it Doc that you charge me hundreds of dollars per hour to fix my body and I only charge you twenty-five dollars per hour to fix your car?" "Because I repair you while you are still running", answered the physician. Do you go running to your physician when you are ill or will you focus instead on creating personal health? Your physician was trained to combat illness. You can train yourself to create health. My point here is to assure you that the body can repair itself while it is running if we create the most favorable conditions eliminating the underlying conditions for most illness.

Let us first begin to learn how we are designed and constructed. As we only begin to explore the wonders and complexity of our body, one cannot dispute that it was created by intelligent design, not evolved on its own.

The best evidence to support creation versus evolution was presented by Dr. Carey Reams in the 1970's and never disproved. Dr. Reams discovered that every living species has an individual frequency that prevents inter breeding between species like man and apes. It is interesting to note that the Bible teaches that all plants and animals have something known as "its own kind". This is repeated in Genesis 1 in verses 11–12, 21, and 24–25. The word "kind" in Hebrew means some form of "sorting out" and was used to prevent various plants and animals from crossing between Kinds. According to Dr. Reams, each kind has a number representing its unique frequency. Species can breed and evolve within their own kind but not into different species. Perhaps more important is Dr. Ream's Biological Theory of Ionization which we discuss later. Frequency will be discussed in the section on energy healing.

The Cell

The basic structural component of anything living (or once living) is the Cell. Nothing is more representative of God's perfect design than a living cell. Recently, we watched a wonderful series called, "Focus on the Family's The Truth Project (R)". Perhaps your church has offered it? The comparison was made that when we look at a complex watch we can see immediately that the watch did not suddenly appear out of nowhere, but was the result of intelligent design. The complexity of a living cell cannot be compared to the technology of even the most complex timepiece. It becomes even more difficult to decipher after factoring in its life force or frequency. The intelligent design of a cell is beyond the comprehension of even the most brilliant minds. It did not just evolve.

Visualize a tiny room with walls, ceiling and floor. The living cell is a self-contained microscopic sized factory. There are many different kinds of cells present in the human body, each kind having a specific function. Cells cluster together in specific forms and shapes in order to make up various body structures. Each cell is surrounded by a cell wall called a Membrane. The Membrane is semi-permeable, that means it selectively allows certain specific substances to enter, like nutrients and certain substances to exit, like manufactured enzymes or waste products.

Inside the wall of the factory are many highly specialized components, which are controlled from a command center that is called the Nucleus. With very powerful optics, each cell can be more minutely examined to reveal tiny components called molecules and even smaller ones called atoms. We even have the capability now to see the DNA, gene structure and even smaller components allowing us to marvel at such a miracle of design.

The fuel to energize our body comes from a combination of combustion and electricity produced in specific cells. Combustion comes from the calories, or heat released by the digestion of our food combined with the oxygen we breathe.

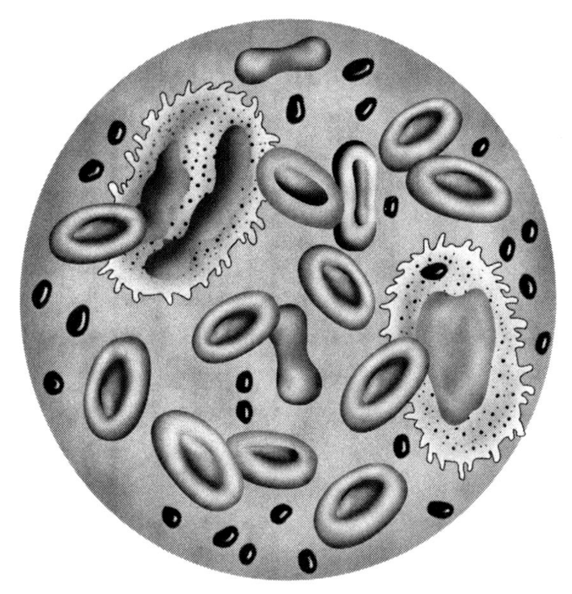

Illus. I: Blood Cell

Electricity comes from charged molecules called **Ions**, which carry a charge we receive from combustion and from the molten iron, magnetic core of the Earth, the Sun and the Universe. Since our body is mostly water with certain essential minerals, like the plates of a car battery, these Ions form electrolytes or charged particles in solution found in every part of our body. Ions can be broken down even further into **Anions** and **Cations** (positive and negative). Our nervous systems of sensory and motor nerves are able to send and receive electrical impulses to and from the brain using these electrolytes. We will discuss this some more in a later section on energy healing.

The miracle of creation comes when a male sperm cell unites with a female egg cell producing a Fertilized Egg. This union almost immediately sets in motion a transformation and multiplication of the original two cells into a cluster which becomes an Embryo—the beginning of new life within the womb of the mother. As the Embryo develops, different cells begin to form the many parts or systems that eventually make up a fully developed infant. Each cell carries the special code that determines our individuality (and our Divinity). Each cell is pre-programmed.

What a miracle to watch how our body responds to a simple skin cut—another example of pre-programming. Nanotechnology—the study of matter on an ultra-small scale—has enabled scientists to observe this amazing occurrence. Special cells are sent to stop the bleeding. Then different cells begin the job of repair until eventually, you cannot see where the cut once was. There are countless processes and elements involved in this one miraculous healing which enables our body to survive—too numerous and scientific for me to get into. However, if just one small link in the chain of events were to be left out or not function properly, then we would bleed to death. Our wondrous Creator has prevented this from occurring.

As we continue to develop and grow until maturity, cells are constantly being replaced as they wear out or become damaged. Many experts believe that every cell in the body is replaced every seven years. Eventually, the built in "time clock of aging" signals the decline of our ability to replace all cells or due to disease or damage, the electricity and combustion shuts down. Life in the body comes to an end.

The Framework or Skeletal System

Certain cells cluster together to form the substance known as bone. Bones are the frameworks of our body. They are like the beams and girders, trusses and joists, rafters and studs of a building. There are several different kinds of bones. Some are long, short, flat and irregular depending on the need. The amazing part is that the bones of our body are connected together in an intricate manner so that we have movement. When two or more surfaces of a bone move against one or more surfaces of another bone we have an articulation or a joint. Cartilage, Ligaments, Muscles, and Tendons hold bones together and also allow a range of motion.

Our bony framework not only gives us shape and form, it also protects vital areas. The skull and spinal bones protect our brain and spinal cord. The rib cage protects the lungs, heart, liver, spleen, kidneys and upper digestive tract. The bowl shape of our pelvis/hip bones protects our lower organs of digestion, elimination, and reproduction.

Even within the bones themselves, are highly specialized cells that produce new red blood cells to replace old ones dying off. Tiny blood vessels carry nutrients to each bone and remove waste. Our bones are similar to a living coral reef.

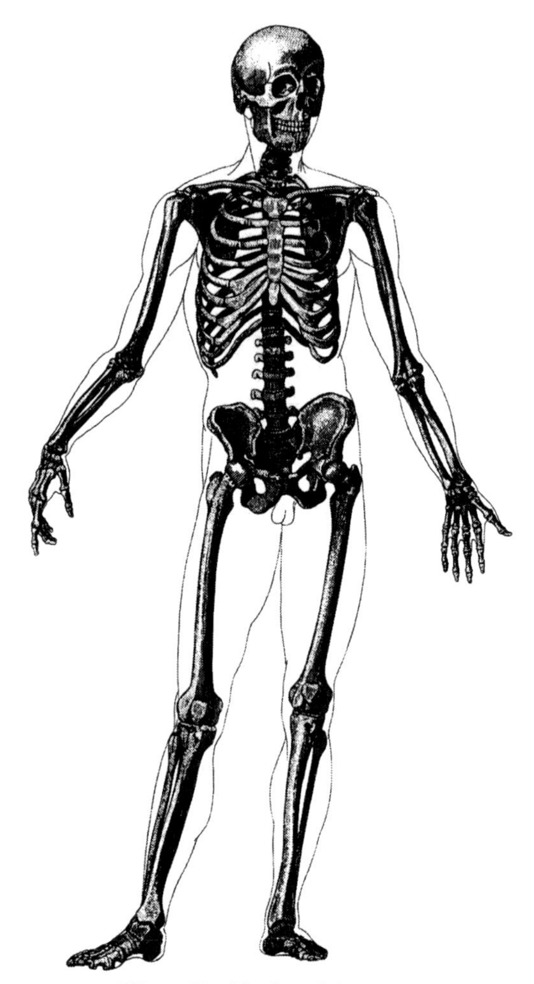

Illus. II: Skeletal System

The most abundant mineral in the body is calcium of which about 99% of it is found in our bones and teeth. In a complex combination with phosphorus, calcium provides rigidity and hardness to our teeth and skeletal system. Besides these two essential minerals, bone building requires other nutrients such as Vitamin D (produced from daily sun exposure), protein (not necessarily from animal sources), Vitamin A and Vitamin C.

Cartilage, Ligaments, Muscles, Tendons

Special cells form special kinds of tissue called **Cartilage**. Cartilage is usually smooth and rubbery. One type of cartilage lines the surfaces of the bones, which rub against each other within a joint. Another type of Cartilage totally surrounds or encapsulates the joint.

One type of **Ligament** is the very strong fibrous band of cells, which bind the bones of a joint together externally. Another type located inside the joint itself, not only connect bone to bone, but also allow movement, such as the knee and hip joints.

Muscles and **Tendons** are highly specialized. Muscles may be long and flat or short and round. They may be voluntary or involuntary, which means that some act on our thoughts and commands and some react from some pre-determined inner program. Muscles are bands of fibers usually beginning and ending in a stronger fiber called a tendon, by which they are attached to a bone. The Muscles act as the pulleys and levers producing motion at the joints. Just look down at your hand as it performs even the simplest task and see what a miracle it is with everything working in balance and harmony.

There are internal muscles not associated with our framework like heart muscles that work in a different way. They are called involuntary muscles and perform their movement automatically, independent of thought, responding to ever changing conditions—more miraculous design.

The bones, muscles, and accompanying fibrous sheaths of our framework form a layer of body armor protecting our vital parts. When the body is alive, all the cells need nutrition and electricity, which comes via the circulatory and nervous systems.

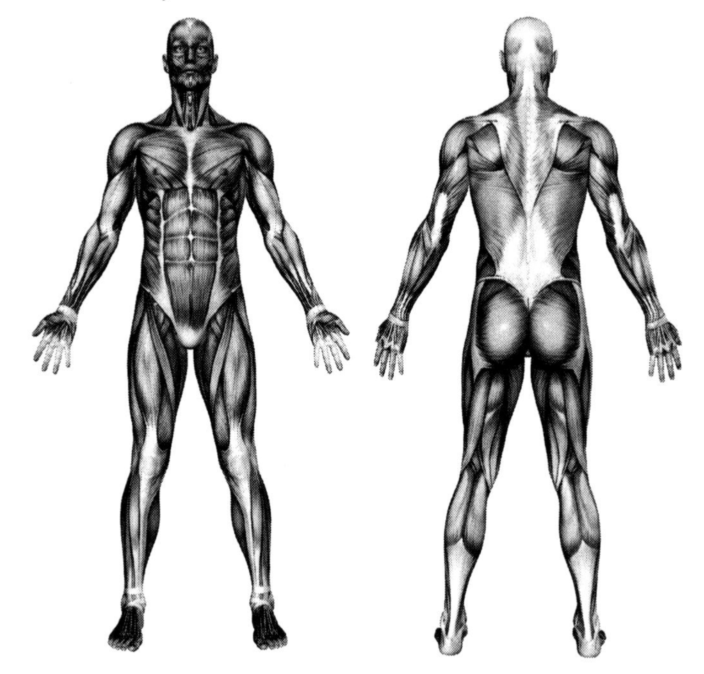

Illus. III: Muscular System

Circulation

Circulation is the process of bringing nutrition to cells and eliminating waste products. There are three systems of circulation in the body with three types of vessels or conveyors called arteries, veins and lymphatic.

Blood is the fluid, consisting of plasma—a clear, yellowish suspension—blood cells, fats, undigested protein, bacteria, viruses and the platelets that aid in clotting. The heart pumps blood through the arteries and veins carrying oxygen and nutrients to and waste materials away from all body tissues.

Illus. IV: Circulation

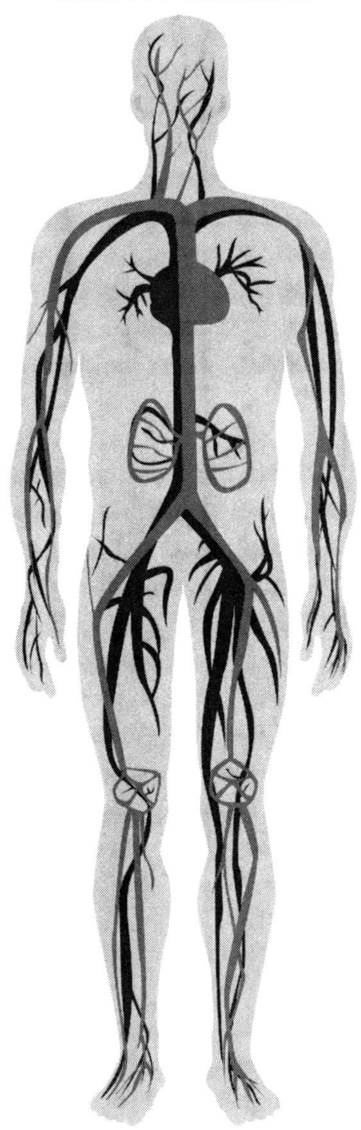

Arteries bring freshly enriched blood from the heart and lungs to every cell. These oxygen enriched blood cells are bright red in color.

Veins return used blood to be re-vitalized. These cells depleted of oxygen are dark red. Veins differ from arteries in that the walls have special valves that open allowing blood to flow towards the heart with each pumping heartbeat but close when the blood falls back between beats. The heart has similar valves.

The pumping action of the **heart** pumps fresh blood as far as your big toe but the heart alone cannot pump the used blood back up again through the veins without some help. It is the squeezing action of our muscles by involuntary contraction and voluntary exercise that assist our heart.

When our legs get out of shape, we put a strain on our heart. Can you see how important exercise is to having a healthy heart?

Lymphatics are the conveyors of a fluid called Lymph that carries waste products from the cells to be shuttled by the blood to the spleen, liver, kidneys, colon and skin for elimination. This system also produces and delivers white blood cells to fight infection and destroy abnormal cells such as cancer cells. The white blood cells are produced in clusters of special cells called nodes as well as produced in the spleen. **Lymph nodes**—of which, there are over six hundred throughout our body—are found in our neck, arm pits, and groin. The lymphatic system is an essential part of our immune system. This is the simplest description of a very complex network.

The lymphatic vessels run parallel to the blood veins in the body. These vessels are filled with a pale fluid called "lymph" that is collected in the space between the cells of the body. These fluids transport nutrients to the cells and then carry the cellular waste back to the blood. Lymph moves slowly under pressure since it depends mostly on the skeletal muscles to squeeze fluid through them. Like veins, lymph vessels have one-way valves and the fluid flows upward through our bodies. Lymph vessels found in the lining of the gastrointestinal tract play an important role in digestion because they transport the fats that we eat for processing.

Did you know that the lymph system is twice the size of our circulatory system? Twice as much lymph as blood is present in our bodies, and we have twice as many lymph vessels as blood vessels. That should speak to the importance of this often overlooked process within our bodies. The lymph system can be thought of as the cellular toxin disposal system—when it is backed-up, it can be life threatening.

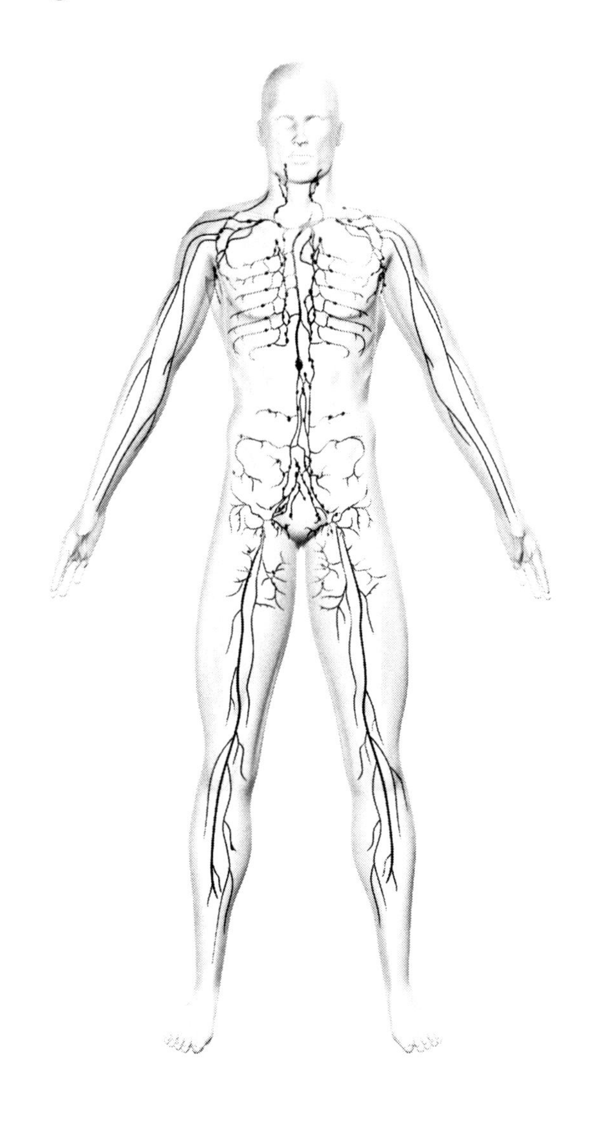

Illus. V: Lymphatic System

The Nervous System

The nervous system consists of the brain, spinal cord and sets of wires or fibers extending from them to all parts of our body called nerves.

The **Brain** is the master computer of our body and has many functions. It consists of sections called lobes each performing specific tasks. The brain requires about 65% of our nutrition and many small blood vessels continually circulate our blood to our brain. Look at the implications of that last statement again.

There are two types of nerves or wires in the body. One type is called **sensory**, which means that it carries sensations back to the brain for interpretation. The other type is called **motor**, which means that they carry impulses from the brain to the voluntary muscles producing motion. Other electrical impulses—from our brain to our internal organs and glands—regulate activity we are not consciously aware of most of the time, referred to as the "autonomic nervous system".

We are an electrical animal, albeit very low voltage and mili-amperage. We are totally hard-wired to every part of our body from the brain and spinal cord. Electrical impulses carried by the nerves activate every cell in our body. Like most electrical objects, we are designed to work best within a certain range or frequency of compatible energy. More about this will be discussed in a future chapter.

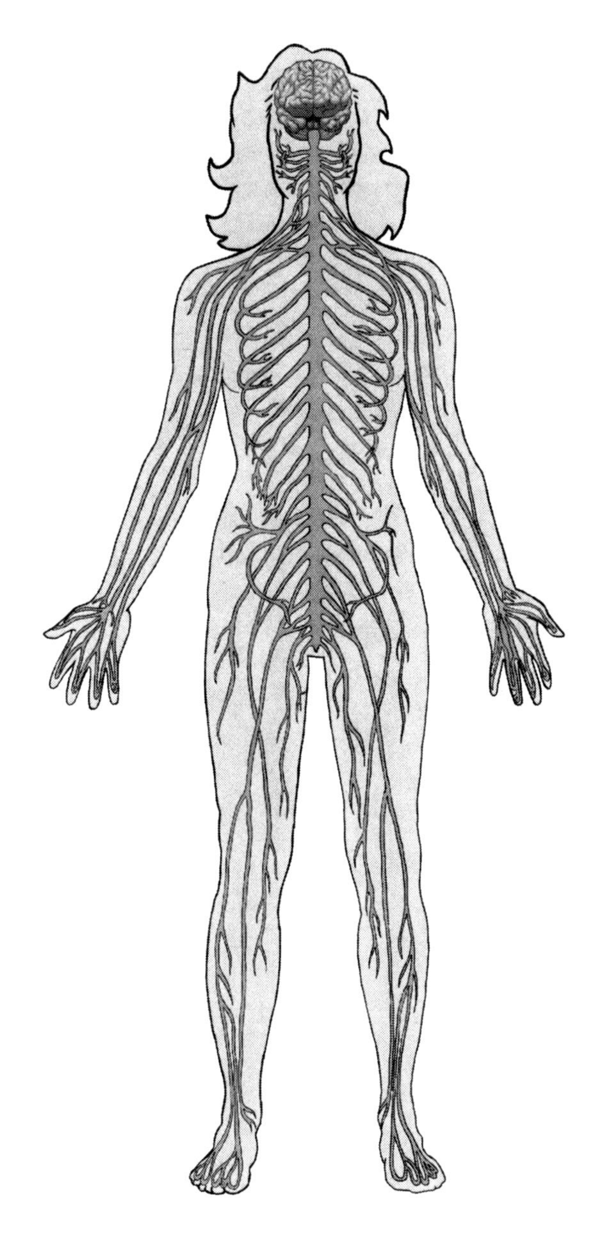

Illus. VI: Nervous System

Organs and Glands

An **Organ** is a specialized group of cells that perform a specific function. A **Gland** is an organ that produces a secretion to be used elsewhere in the body. Some may be both organ and gland. Confusing? Let's look at some examples of each.

We usually think of the following as organs: **Liver** (both organ and gland), **Lungs**, **Heart**, **Kidneys**, **Stomach**, **Spleen**, **Pancreas** (both organ and gland), **Large** and **Small Intestine**.

The following are considered glands: **Pituitary**, **Thyroid**, and **Parathyroid**, **Thymus**, **Adrenal**, **Pancreas**, **Sebaceous**, **Salivary**, **Gallbladder**, **Ovaries**, **Mammary Glands, Prostate**, and **Testicles**.

ORGANS…

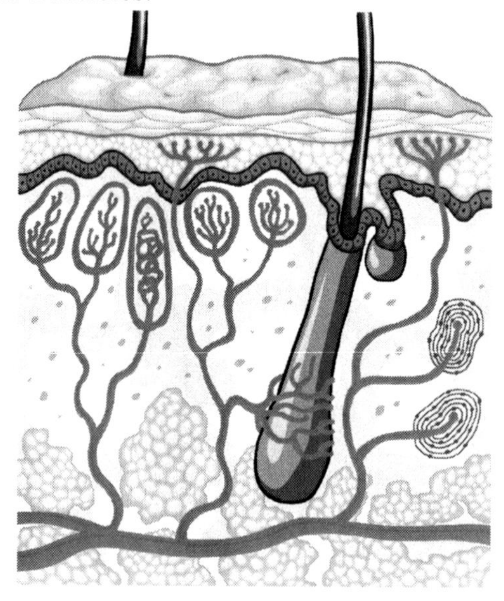

Illus. VI-a: Skin and Fat

Skin, our outer covering, is the largest "organ" of the body. An organ is a specialized part of our body—a cluster of cells that performs a specific function. Most all of our organs are internal except for our skin. External skin is not only our first line of defense but also acts as a semi-permeable membrane that exchanges gases and liquids. Skin has several layers. The outermost layer has sensory nerves, hair and minute openings called pores for respiration and perspiration and it is always shedding dead cells. The inner layers contain blood vessels, nerves and fat cells.

Fat cells insulate our body and are storage for many unused calories and residual toxins.

Naturally, the skin being the most visible organ of the body that can absorb substances such as nutrients and toxins into the body and release substances out from the body, it is the most obvious indication of a body out of balance. It changes color, texture and forms all kinds of skin eruptions and rashes, all indicative of a body out of balance. Skin problems should mainly be treated from the inside out and not just on the surface. However, the sloughing off of dead skin cells, discussed later in Chapter 3, aids this natural process of absorption and elimination.

The **Liver** is our second largest organ, after skin, but is our largest organ of digestion. It is located behind our lower right rib cage. The liver is thought to be the only organ that can regenerate itself. It secretes bile to aid in the digestion of fat and protein, filters and stores toxins from the blood and produces various enzymes which not only help extract nutrients from food like iron and vitamin A and D but also enzymes that assist in wound healing and prevent blood clotting in vessels.

Dr. N. W. Walker, recognized worldwide as one of the most authoritative students of life, health and nutrition, speaks of the liver in his book *The Vegetarian Guide to Diet and Salads* as "Created by nature to withstand, on an average, about 40–50 years of abuse after birth before perceptible and usually uncomfortable disintegration begins." So it stands to reason that if we do not over abuse our liver we would be extending the health of our body as we age.

The **Lungs** located in our upper chest cavity exchange fresh air and used air through our mouth and nose. They consist of two spongy like sacs that exchange mostly carbon dioxide and oxygen in the blood by means of many tiny arteries and veins.

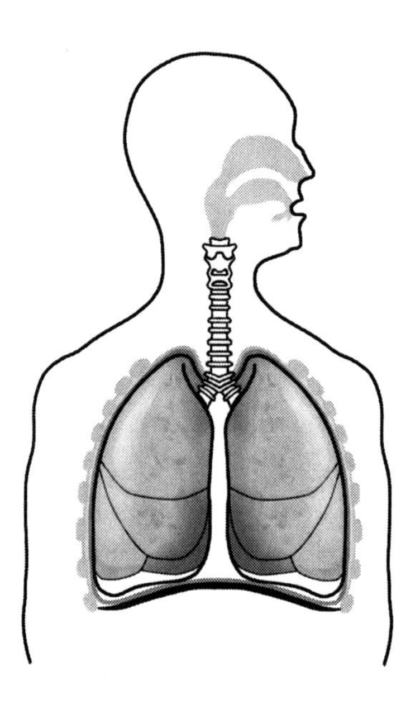

Illus. VI-b: Lungs

The **Heart** is a four-chambered pumping muscle located in our mid-chest cavity that circulates our blood and is the epicenter of our spiritual being. Since it is the force behind our circulation, it enables the blood to bring needed nutrients to every cell of our body and remove the excess and waste products.

The **Kidneys** are a pair, one on either side of the lower, rear abdominal cavity, which control water balance and filter the blood of certain impurities. They help to regulate pH levels, electrolytes and actual fluid volume.

The **Stomach** is the main sac-like organ of digestion located in the lower abdominal cavity. Digestion really begins in the mouth with proper chewing of food into mush before swallowing and then the stomach secretes other enzymes to further break down food for our nutritional needs. It churns and mixes foods for short time periods if the food is easy to digest, like fresh fruit. A fatty meal takes longer.

The **Spleen** is a large organ located on the left side behind our lower rib cage that aids in the removal of waste from the lymph system and produces white blood cells called lymphocytes.

The **Pancreas** is a long gland/organ located behind the stomach. Special cells produce insulin and glycogen—hormones that regulates our blood sugar. Other cells produce Pancreatin, an enzyme that aids in the digestion of protein and fat that the pancreas secretes into the small intestine.

The **Small Intestine** connects to the stomach and is the next organ of digestion. It is many feet long and consists of specialized segments, each one designed to break down food into usable nutrients that it absorbs and passes on thru the circulation in the walls. When we can visualize the complexity of our lower intestinal tract it becomes clear that there are many bends and kinks where debris can accumulate.

The **Colon** or large intestine begins in our lower right abdomen just above where our appendix is, or is not as the case may be. This is the juncture where the small intestine and the ascending colon extend upward to our right rib cage near our liver then across or transversely to our left side near our spleen and descend down to our rectum.

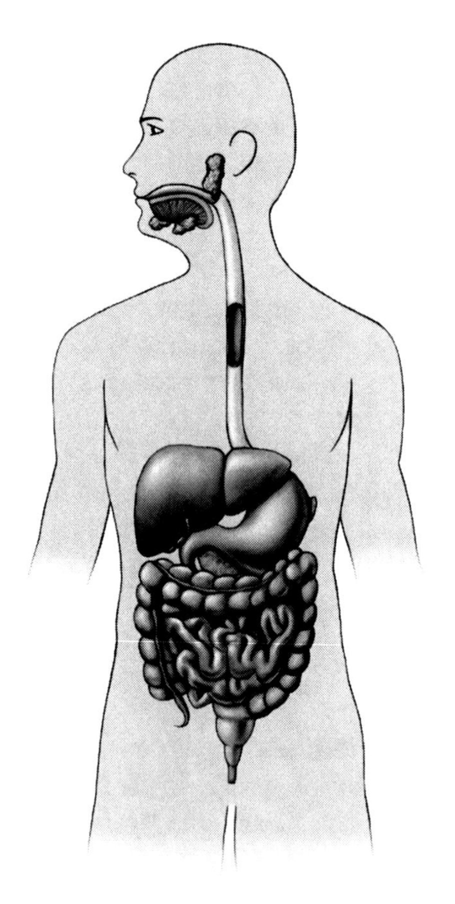

Illus. VI-c: Digestive System

The colon is the sewer system of the body and is partly responsible for much illness and disease due to poor function.

The **Appendix,** located at the bottom of the ascending colon, is considered a "vestigial" or rudimentary organ (a sign of something that no longer exists) by modern medicine and is routinely surgically removed when it becomes inflamed (Appendicitis). When the ascending colon becomes sluggish in eliminating waste the appendix acts as an overflow and warning valve. Thus, inflammation is an indication that something is terribly wrong above and needs correction. Removal of the appendix does not eliminate the cause.

GLANDS…

The **Pituitary** is considered to be the "master gland", as it regulates many other glands called endocrine, which pass their secretions directly into the bloodstream. It is located at the base of the brain. It secretes hormones that regulate growth and the regulation of other glands such as the **Thyroid** which regulates caloric burn and is located on either side of our windpipe. The **Thymus** regulates our immunity and is located at the top and behind the breastbone while the **Adrenals,** located on top of each kidney, secrete adrenalin for quick energy and cortisone for inflammation.

Other glands are the **Gallbladder** located under the liver, which stores bile to digest fat and to lubricate the intestines. The **Ovaries** in females, located in the lower abdomen, produce eggs for reproduction and hormones for body regulation. The female breasts or **Mammary Glands** are responsible for milk production for the newborn and regulation of body temperature and hormonal balance in the adult. The **Testicles** in men located in a sac below the penis, produce sperm for reproduction and hormones for body regulation. The **Prostate** is located just under the bladder, behind the penis. It controls urinary flow and with the sperm from the testicles produces the fluid called semen.

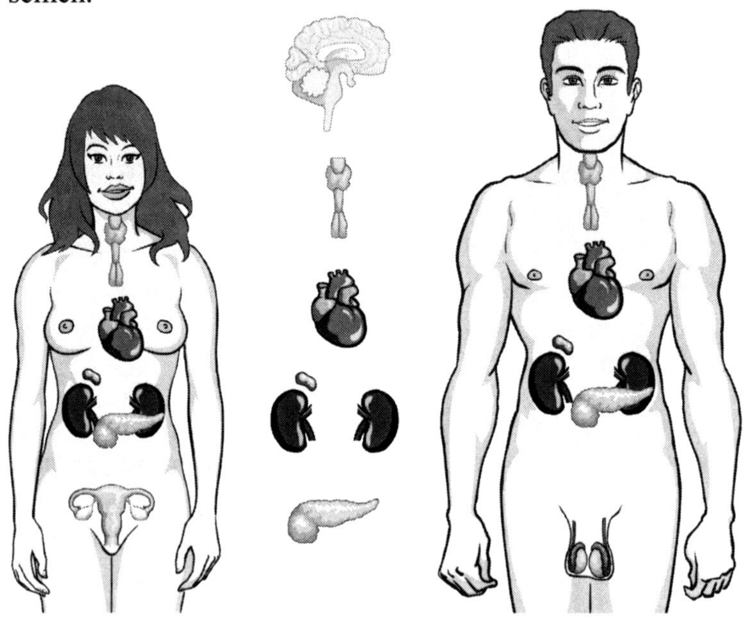

Illus. VI-d: Endocrine System

Sebaceous glands release sweat and are located almost wherever there is hair. **Salivary** glands are located above and below the gums of the mouth and release the first digestive enzymes from proper chewing of food. Saliva contains amylase, which breaks down carbohydrates and lysozyme which kills bacteria.

We have just briefly described how our body is constructed and designed to function. Can you imagine how complex our physical being is and how wondrously it works? Only a masterful intelligence beyond our own comprehension—namely, God—could have devised such perfection.

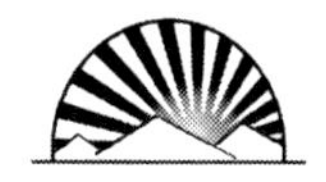

Chapter Two: **Why We Get Sick**

With very few exceptions we ourselves, are the cause of almost every illness. How, Why, What, you say? Our diets, lifestyles, thoughts and behavior patterns create most wellness or illness. We may not be born with good health and immunity due to what we received from our mother during development and infancy, but:

The actual cause of illness is...the body is out of balance.

Balance is a miraculous condition when everything is in perfect harmony and functioning as it was designed. In medical terms this is named "homeostasis". Balance is necessary not only of our body but, also for a "see-saw (teeter totter)", a skyscraper, an airplane, a tree, and a flower, the Sun, Moon, Stars and the entire Universe. As we look around us, if what we see is out of balance, it would either fall apart or die.

How does our body become out of balance? The answer is, many ways. Jesus told us that "No man can serve two masters…." (Mat 6:24) We cannot keep our temple pure and continually poison ourselves. The body can be out of balance chemically, nutritionally, physically, emotionally, and spiritually. In reality there are no clear cut distinctions—there is an interweaving and overlapping as one imbalance affects another. Let us explore them one at a time.

A CHEMICAL IMBALANCE is usually multi-faceted…

Without clean air, clean water or clean food, we would not stay alive very long.

Today, our air, water and food have all, to some degree, become contaminated. The contaminations are called toxins and "Toxemia" is the condition when our body becomes overloaded with harmful poison. Some toxins are actually produced within the body because of the putrefaction and fermentation of undigested animal protein.

Without clean air we would perish in just a few minutes. We tend to take air for granted. It is composed of many gases—all within a specific range of content—that keep us alive. Were someone to back a diesel truck up to your house and attach a hose from the engine exhaust pipe into your window, you would soon be gasping for clean air. The balance would be thrown off. The same would be true were someone to dump gasoline in your drinking water, you would soon be very sick.

The contamination of our air, water and food supply is happening in much more subtle ways as well as some obvious ways but what are we doing about it? If we are to be concerned about the outside air—as many of us are today—then we need to be equally concerned about the inside air where we live, work and socialize. Molds, viruses and bacteria flourish in closed-in spaces that do not get any natural sunlight or fresh outside air. Air conditioning ducts, carpeting, drapes and basements are breeding grounds for all kinds of microscopic "nasties" that make us sick. More and more we have insulated ourselves from our natural surroundings and chosen instead to confine ourselves to central heating and air-conditioning environments. This situation is tolerable just as long as those responsible practice a high level of maintenance by cleaning ducts and drapes and carpets, etc., on a regular basis and letting fresh air and light in whenever possible—but how often do you think this is being done? I have stopped going to movie theaters years ago since I believe they are the unhealthiest place to be in. Even after being cleaned these closed-in spaces then expose us to the residual chemicals left behind.

As a society, we typically give the responsibility for our air, water and food to others. As long as we fail to take any action to prevent contamination, we will undoubtedly continue to have chemical imbalances in our bodies. Most people have many unnatural chemicals (usually man made) in their bodies that lead to illness. These toxins come into our food via farm chemicals and processing and from polluted air and water to name but a few sources. We also produce some toxins of our own from the putrefaction and fermentation of undigested animal protein. Other sources might be mercury dental fillings and the poisons used in dental root canal procedures. Good personal detective work is necessary to reveal what irritants are present in your cleaning agents, toothpaste, deodorants, soaps and shampoos, air fresheners, fabric softeners and so on and so on. We are being accosted with these harmful substances more and more. Chemicals can be poisonous to our body over time and illness may not be felt immediately after exposure. Poisons that are mainly stored in the fat, liver, spleen and colon, eventually reach anywhere in your body via the blood. This attack on our health will not end as long as we continue to buy into the latest procedure, service, product, or any modern day convenience—that is more profit driven than concerned with maintaining our health, especially when it comes to our food.

There is another chemical imbalance in our bodies that is terribly neglected and it is that most people have an imbalance in their pH or acid/alkaline balance. When we are too acidic we become ill, which results in calcium being pulled from the bones and teeth in order to buffer the over acid condition. The result is osteoporosis in the mature and cavities in the teeth of the young. Cancer, arthritis and many more illnesses are enhanced when our ph is too acidic. This is a critical component of the wellness equation and much more will be discussed in the chapter on diet.

There are often imbalances in sodium and potassium, in calcium and magnesium and many other minerals due to the degrading of our soil quality resulting in lower food quality—thus lacking the sustenance we need to stay healthy. When we are not getting the nutrition that should come from our food, it is no wonder that the marketing of herbs and supplements is a huge profit making industry. I used to think that vitamins and supplements were for folks with special needs and/or those folks who couldn't or wouldn't eat balanced diets. Now, the manufacturers harp on the fact that your food may not be what it used to be. Processed and refined foods eliminate what value remains and then try to put it back artificially. Our bodies, however, aren't being fooled and often can not break down and utilize these added elements so they end up having to be eliminated or stored where they don't belong.

The water you drink or that is contained in beverages could be a source of a chemical imbalance. On Sept. 25, 2009, it was reported by the Associated Press that its investigation had revealed that contaminates—such as lead, pesticides, herbicides and many other toxins—were discovered in the drinking water of public and private schools of small towns and inner cities in all fifty states. Water safety violations for our school children have gone largely unmonitored for the past decade. Schools relying on well water in the California farm belt were especially affected. There are other reasons for this besides pesticides and this same tainted water has also shown up in homes and businesses forcing people to turn to bottled water instead. However, don't just make safe assumptions about that expensive bottled water you just bought. Here are some questions you should ask yourself:

- Where does my water come from?
- How is it being filtered or processed?
- Is anything being added to my drinking water?
- Has it been tested to see if it will do me harm?
- Is the plastic bottle contaminating the water?

The immoral, unhealthy and profit-driven practices of industries have definitely polluted our once clean rivers, lakes and streams. Some municipalities actually recycle used or unclean water through large filtering plants. Do you know where your own water comes from? How safe is it really? If you live in a large metropolitan area, your water supply, being from only one source, is critical to your good health. It is important to use an installed or stand alone filtering system of your own before drinking rather than relying on whatever comes out of your tap. And if you live in a rural area where farming is done, your well or spring water could very well be contaminated from herbicides, pesticides and chemicals that are carried in the air or seep down and travel underground. If we are to accept responsibility for our health and the health of others and the health of our planet, we must keep in mind that we all live downstream or downwind from someone else. This means that what we do affects our neighbor and what our neighbor does affects us. Are we not heeding the Lord's second greatest commandment? Jesus said, "Thou shalt love thy neighbor as thyself" (Mat.22:39). To be a good Christian or Jew or any righteous person today means standing up for what is right and being responsible for what is happening around you and how it affects your neighbor.

Besides the effects of toxic water, another much overlooked cause of a chemical imbalance is simply the fact that we do not consume nearly enough water for all our bodily systems to function normally. Water is very much needed to keep everything moving, flush out waste, produce an electrical current for energy, and to dissolve excess salts that can accumulate and cause heart attacks. Many symptoms, as common as a headache or constipation can be relieved by consuming more water. I can not stress often enough the importance of drinking half your body weight in ounces of pure water per day.

There are unseen dangers affecting our body chemistry…

Non-visible radiation produces chemical changes within our body. Some non-visible wave lengths of energy given off by man made and natural sources can affect us negatively. A microwave oven, for instance, gives off small amounts of external radiation but reputable scientific studies done in Sweden show that negative blood changes also occur after consuming "micro-waved" food. Soon after these clinical studies, conducted by Dr. Hans Hertel, were made public the hammer of authority came down on him. A powerful trade organization in Sweden forced the hand of government to issue a "gag" order. The threat of loss of revenue from diminished sales of microwave ovens weighed heavier in the courts than any threat that was shown to exist to the health of the consumers. Governments don't always have our best interest at heart even though that is the role that God designed them to play. We, as consumers must become better informed and not rely on popular opinion or the manipulative influences that play on our weaknesses. Not everything faster and easier is better.

Simply put, here is how a microwave oven works: The cooking heat is generated from friction within the cells as water molecules are torn apart and structurally deformed thereby impairing quality. Conventional heating of food transfers the heat from without to within by convection and has been shown to produce the least amount of structural change to the food that is heated as compared with microwaves.

Other studies have made similar claims pointing to the ill effects of these modern conveniences. In 1989, Young Families, the Minnesota Extension Services of the University of Minnesota, announced on the radio that heating baby's bottle was not recommended in a microwave. First, it was because the liquid in the bottle becomes extremely hot although the outside may remain cool to the touch and a build up of steam in the enclosed container could cause it to explode. Secondly, they said that slight changes to the milk or formula occur while depleting nutrients and destroying some protective properties of breast milk. Another study appearing in the journal *Pediatrics* (Vol. 89, No. 4, April 1992) indicated that microwaving human milk—even at a low setting—can destroy some of its important disease-fighting capabilities…and there have been others, all pertaining to breast milk. More studies are obviously needed but apparently are not being funded, I believe, because they go against the establishment. The microwave oven industry has basically only been held accountable to insure that the dangerous microwaves were being contained and not to what extent they affected the quality of the food being heated inside the oven.

Harmful microwaves can be found outside of the kitchen as well. The jury may still be out on the issue of harm from cell phones, but I am convinced that we receive harmful microwaves to our brain when we hold a cell phone close to our head. Many reports have come out about the higher occurrence of brain cancer and tumors felt to be the result of the increased use of cell phones. We often think to ourselves that "what we cannot see cannot hurt us" but can we really rely on this logic today? X-rays and atomic radiation are also non-visible and harmful to people.

There are full-body computed tomography scans that you sometimes see at the mall that should be avoided. CT scans deliver a dose of radiation 50–200 times that of a conventional x-ray. Studies have shown that they often give a false positive resulting in the need for further testing. If your doctor orders a non-emergency CT scan (say, to investigate headaches), ask if a radiation-free ultrasound or an MRI can be used instead and stick to shopping when at the mall.

In the opinion of many reputable experts, mammograms expose women to harmful low dose radiation. I wrote the following commentary regarding mammograms in 1995 and it was published in The Free Weekly of Fayetteville, AR.:

FREE MAMMOGRAMS?

> After many years of advocating annual mammograms, the Medical Industry is now advertising Free Mammograms...and yet breast cancer is on the rise. The profitable business of medical testing utilizing mammograms, catscans, MRI and x-ray can transmit harmful radiation which induces cancer according to many prestigious scientists outside the USA. The American Medical Industry needs their own devised methods of testing to provide constant customers for the myriad of profitable procedures like needle biopsies, lumpectomies, lymphnodectomies and mastectomies—all of which can

spread cancer and only treat symptoms not causes—and yet breast cancer is on the rise.

Monopolistic, political and legal manipulating industries like corporate medicine, pharmaceutical, insurance, banking, chemical and agriculture all synergistically profit from the present business of cancer.

The proven methods for curing cancer consist of rejecting western medicine, pharmaceutical drugs, chemicals, commercial food and lifestyle, while choosing instead to take personal responsibility for self-healing. The proven cures and methods employed by thousands since the 1920s are never publicized or taught except by medical revolutionaries and are not utilized except by people who either have run the gamut of orthodox medicine or have the fortitude and intelligence to change their personal habits and lifestyles—rejecting the pressures of peers and current socio/economic trends.

Beware of Free Mammograms or any exposure to radiation however benign the sales-pitch because radiation is cumulative in our bodies from utero and like a time bomb eventually causes destruction—more so than most other toxins.

The human body has the ability to heal itself unless it is overwhelmed with toxins. The solution is simple and not profitable. We all need to know from birth how to detoxify our bodies and maintain a healthful lifestyle.

I stand by this same opinion today. Nothing has changed…

Microwaves (not just ovens, but data transmission), electronic door openers, cell phones, radar guns and high voltage power lines are just a few types of energy that can produce negative chemical changes in our bodies. However, not all forms of energy are bad for us in fact, everything is composed of energy. Imagine if you will what it might be like to "bathe in a rainbow". To our eyes there are seven colors that are visible in a rainbow. They are red, orange, yellow, green, blue, lavender and violet. This rainbow of colors is very compatible with our body. The natural, vibrational energy of these colors is healing and will be discussed more in a section on energy healing.

A NUTRITIONAL IMBALANCE is due to poor dietary habits…

The necessary vitamins and minerals required to keep us healthy should come from our food. I strongly believe this often quoted statement, "Our medicine should be our food and our food should be our medicine." As previously mentioned under "chemical imbalances", this often may not be the case. Knowing where and how our food is grown will help us to make better choices but more about this later in Chapter Four.

Proper portioning of food at each meal between vegetables, proteins and grains maintains good health. Processed and refined foods should be eliminated. Sugar consumption is more addicting and more harmful to the body than any so called dangerous drug, even heroin. Too much protein, especially of animal origin overtaxes our digestive systems. If you have a serious illness at this time, then you need to understand that the more you can limit the body's energy spent on digestion, the more energy the body can direct towards healing. Too much protein also greatly upsets the acid/alkaline balance—which was previously mentioned under chemical imbalances—producing a highly acidic environment in the body that is very conducive to the growth of cancer.

Today, most soils are lacking in essential mineral nutrients and so are the foods grown in them. Even if we make the best food choices the food may be lacking in essential nutrients due to mis-management of our soils—more about this in the chapter on agriculture. However, lack of minerals is a prime cause of illness.

Dr. Carey A. Reams, whom I referred to earlier in my journey to wellness, confirms in his book *Choose Life or Death* saying, "Ill health does not result from one single event in our daily life, but a combination of things, plus lack of minerals in our dietary program."

The ill effects of a body overgrown with yeast and/or parasites…

There is a war going on in your body at this very moment. Not only against foreign invaders which come from without like bacteria and viruses but also there is a war within our body playing host to friendly and un-friendly organisms. Yeast or Candida and parasites of numerous species reside inside you at this very moment. Your ability to resist illness decreases when the "bad guys" overwhelm the "good guys" who are living on the same block. A proliferation of yeast and parasites comes from a dietary imbalance and has been linked to almost every serious illness.

Parasites not only come from raw food—especially sushi—or improperly cooked food but are also found in cured deli meats such as pork and the infamous ham sandwich. Swine are very prone to harboring tape worms and trichinella worms that can cause serious illness, even death, when left unchecked in humans. These meats are often stored in a refrigerator for an extended period of time giving bacteria time to flourish as well. Use caution when selecting what and where to eat and spare your self from a whole lot of parasites. You can't beat cleanliness and fresh ingredients when choosing a restaurant.

Bad bacteria or yeast overgrowth, also referred to as “Candida” is a problem, I would say, existing in most everyone today due to our insatiable craving of sweets and baked goods made with baker’s yeast. Yeast connected disorders are affecting people of all ages ranging from fatigue, headache and depression to a myriad of chronic and severe illness such as asthma, multiple sclerosis and even cancer.

Addressing these two imbalances is an essential part of our cleansing programs. These subjects will also be further addressed in the chapter on diet.

A PHYSICAL IMBALANCE can be hereditary or acquired…

There may be a birth defect, an injury or a loss of function due to aging, disease, lack of use, or exercise. Any physical imbalance puts more strain on some other part of us to take up the slack. For instance when your abdominal muscles get out of shape and you begin to sag in the gut, your low back muscles will begin to hurt because of the extra load placed upon them to support your spine. This is a very common symptom of a physical imbalance called overweight. All the systems of your normal body functions have to work harder.

Let me give you an example. Suppose I came up to you and thrust an 80–100 pound bag of cement into your arms and said, “Carry that around with you for twenty-four hours”. Could you do it, probably not? Yet many people are that much over weight and more. But if I handed you a small ¼ pound (4 ounce) bag of cement to carry around for twenty-four hours, you could do that easily. Suppose the next day, I gave you another ¼ pound and again every day for a year? There is very good chance that *you* would gradually adjust to the excess weight but your body really doesn't.

Obesity is an obvious problem today that I see wherever I go. You really do not need a statistician to prove to you the severity of this condition in our present day culture. It is all around us and it is especially alarming in our youth. This is a symptom of a lifestyle and a society that is way out of balance. Our youth should be strong and healthy and leading active lives. Instead, they are developing diseases earlier and earlier in life that usually only show up much later in life due to years of abuse and neglect for their body's needs. Our schools contribute to physical imbalances by forcing students to sit for long periods on ill-designed furniture. As we age we lose that youthful exuberance to go out to play. What a crime it is that our youth, today, are losing it too because they have become computer game junkies instead or, worse yet, motor scooter or four-wheeler junkies. Even our youth have mostly given up walking. Couple that with junk food and you have a recipe for premature illness.

What we need is for all ages, both young and old, to get out together and play more. Find something physical to do in the fresh air and a little daily sunshine, enjoy nature and reconnect with the wonders of God. We also need to develop a daily exercise routine to restore or maintain fitness. Posture needs to be taught in childhood. I'll say more about this in the chapter on stress.

AN EMOTIONAL IMBALANCE can be the most serious imbalance…

I consider this kind of imbalance to be the most serious mainly because it is, more often than not, the hardest to correct. There are many influences that can trigger an emotional imbalance….

There is an old saying, "What man can conceive he can achieve". Our thoughts are the seeds of both positive and negative fruit. "For as he thinketh in his heart, so *is* he", states Proverbs 23:7. We can literally create our own reality with our thoughts. Illness sometimes brings rewards that we may be seeking, like getting more attention. An acceptable way of committing suicide is to contract a severe illness like cancer. In fact, there seems to be a thread of similarity among most cancer sufferers. This thread is that at some time in their lives, the person with cancer became extremely negative to such an extent that they programmed themselves (subconsciously) with the thoughts that life was not worth living any more. To discover the root of such thoughts, to own them and to release them is part of the process of healing.

A program that has proven very beneficial in releasing emotional stress is casually referred to as "Potters" of the Potter's Institute. The Fountain of Life Church, of which we are a member here in Belize, has been very active in bringing this workshop into this area for people who have emotional and spiritual healing to do or just want to renew their personal relationship with God. It takes place over four days and it enables students to cleanse themselves and be healed of hurts from their past. During this time, God reveals to them how much they have allowed themselves to be defeated by holding on to past offenses and wounds of the heart. People who have taken this course have made an important effort towards changing their lives for the better. We must do our part in order for God to step in and to do His part. When we bare ourselves fully to the Lord, He hears us and brings us comfort. Most of us hold on to our ailments perhaps because we are not ready to fully surrender. Proverbs 14:30 (NKJV) says:

> *A calm and undisturbed mind and heart are the life and health of the body, but envy, jealousy, and wrath are like rottenness of the bones.*

Not everyone is blessed with having grown up in a non-dysfunctional, wholesome and loving family home being taught good Christian morals. Each of us can probably recall some hurtful experience when words or actions left an emotional scar. Children can especially be mean to other children when they have not been taught how to handle their own feelings or a particular situation wisely. Just today, I read in the news that studies now show that obesity in children does not cause low self-esteem but rather, low self-esteem causes obesity. I believe this is true for all ages. How often is someone likely to push down painful or angry feelings by stuffing themselves with food? What everyone needs is a feeling of being loved, having self-worth and having some meaningful work or purpose in life. Once we realize that our experience of this world alone is not all that there is and that we can overcome all things in Christ, we can be lifted up and motivated to live a life of service which brings great joy and satisfaction. Paul writes in Philippians 2:4 (NKJV):

> *Let each of you esteem and look upon and be concerned for not [merely] his own interests, but also each for the interests of others.*

We were created in God's image for love—to love and to be loved. Even if you do not profess to be a Christian, you would probably agree that we all have a need for love and when we do not receive enough genuine love we lose our own capacity to love others. When this happens, we may begin to seek love in all the wrong places by acting rebelliously and/or by adopting destructive habits or we can become compulsive in seeking attention by over-achieving and being too demanding of others. In either case, it leads to a person's life and body being out of balance. Relationships suffer greatly until we can get in touch with the unfulfilled need (s) and learn to love.

Rose has been watching a nine part DVD series called "Experiencing the Father's Embrace" presented by long time pastor, Jack Frost. He emphasizes that, "A need not met results in an illness and a need met results in wellness." I couldn't agree with him more, whether it is a physical or an emotional need we must get back into balance by discovering the missing link. All too often, people have either mother or father issues of one kind or another that they are still harboring. According to Jack Frost, who speaks from his own difficult life experiences, if we can reconnect with the painful and disappointing events of our childhood and then process them through a heart-felt embrace of our Father God's unconditional love, we can be healed and develop healthy relationships. The key is to stay centered in God's love and not to allow oneself to go adrift.

The Bible is full of practical advice for righteous human behavior. By consciously striving to build each other up through our words and actions we can prevent emotional strife. However, Pastor Jack makes another good point when he claims that you can not be a good father or mother until you have first become a good son or daughter and completely healed your emotional past. We have to break the chain that binds us to generations of dysfunctional relationships. Once we can accomplish this, setting a good example for our children goes a long way in teaching love and respect for others. This is the foundation of healthy relationships in all areas of our life and helps us to cope in times of conflict.

But, perhaps you are experiencing a conflict of another kind? Many people have developed split personalities. There is the person that goes to work everyday to earn enough money only so they can afford to do what he or she really desires to do. Money is the driving influence in their life and not the satisfaction that comes from doing their best at what they are being called to do now. This type of person usually hates to get up in the morning and face another day. If you do not greet each day with the joyful anticipation of a small child, you need to re-evaluate your priorities.

There is also an old 1944 song that I am very fond of singing by Johnny Mercer and Harold Arlen, made popular by Bing Crosby that says, "You've got to accentuate the positive, eliminate the negative, latch on to the affirmative, don't mess with Mr. In-between".

Finally, we have the emotional imbalance caused by stress. We develop stress from an inability to function normally due to improper nutrition, loss of sleep, and lack of exercise—all affecting our mental capabilities and our emotions. This in combination with financial mis-management and worries affects our relationships at home and at work. It is easy to see how all of these imbalances tend to overlap each other and influence our state of wellness.

All too often, we do not heed the words of God through Paul (Phil.4:6) when he says, "Be careful for nothing (do not be anxious about anything); but in everything by prayer and supplication (humble, earnest petition) with thanksgiving let your requests be made known unto God." Worry does nothing but to create more stress. Throughout the day it helps to talk to your Heavenly Father and give things over to Him that you really have no control over anyway and remember to keep thanking Him for handling them.

A SPIRITUAL IMBALANCE comes from not being a co-creator of our purpose for existence with God.

It also comes from holding on to "un-forgiveness" and/or having our priorities become confused with what is unimportant and not being able to identify for ourselves what is really important. I am a teacher not a preacher. Sometimes there is a very fine line between the two. It is my mission to encourage you to "go within" and seek the Holy Spirit as your guide. Pray to God first in the name of Jesus, and then take a step or two in His direction by changing to be a better servant of the Lord. We carry many "strongholds" in our mind that can silently eat away at us by replacing healthy, positive thoughts with negative ones —just like a cancer that destroys healthy tissue and replaces it with infectious growths. One of these strongholds is un-forgiveness.

The Bible shows us many examples of strong character and faith in God. For instance, Joseph endured many hardships as a slave and a prisoner due to the actions of his brothers. However, he held fast to God's promise to him in a dream and most importantly, never bore any resentment nor allowed his circumstances or the opinions of others to beset him. Paul, while on trial before Festus expressed this same sentiment in Acts 24:16: "And herein do I exercise myself, to have always a conscience void of offense toward God, and toward men."

How I came to understand the healing of forgiveness...

Before there was a "Bible", there were scrolls of parchment, papyrus and sheepskin that contained the Laws, Testimonies and Prayers of the children of Israel. The Torah was the ceremonial scroll, the Talmud was the document of Laws and the Kaballa was the record of mysticism. Every Hebrew home had a Siddur, which was a document of prayers for every occasion from birth to death. When printing became available, every family had a bound Siddur which they brought to synagogue as the prayer book.

Jesus, a Hebrew named Yeshua, was born and grew up in this culture. He studied Hebrew for His Bar-Mitzvah—a ceremony of manhood at age thirteen when Jewish youths are recognized to have earned the right to read from the Torah at the synagogue. He learned the sacred prayers and sang the ancient melodies, hymns and chants of Judaism.

Jews were not a forgiving people throughout their history until Jesus, at age thirty, began to teach the Gospel of Forgiveness by Word and Deed. Some of the Jews were paying attention but not nearly enough, as the Bible reveals. There are very few examples of forgiveness in the Old Testament. The one which most often comes to mind is that of Joseph who forgave his brothers when they were in time of famine. (Gen 50:17). God was pictured in those days as a more vengeful and unforgiving Father. Even now and throughout history, Jews and other minority cultures seem to have assumed the role of a persecuted people. The

Holocaust and other forms of genocide produce un-forgiveness

Un-forgiveness is a sickness that permeates the entire body and produces illness. Jesus knew that and there are many references to forgiveness in the New Testament. The most memorable story to me is the one of Jesus forgiving the soldiers that were nailing Him to the Cross. My first lesson in forgiveness was learning the Lord's Prayer as in Luke 11:2-4:

> *When ye pray, say, Our Father which art in heaven, Hallowed be thy name. Thy Kingdom come. Thy will be done, as in heaven, so in earth. Give us day by day our daily bread. And forgive us our sins; for we also forgive everyone that is indebted to us. And lead us not into temptation; but deliver us from evil.*

But the most powerful teaching to me is the one in Luke 17:3-4:

> *Take heed to yourselves: If thy brother trespass against thee, rebuke him; and if he repent, forgive him. And if he trespass against thee seven times in a day, and seven times in a day turn again to thee, saying, I repent; thou shalt forgive him.*

Forgiveness is liberating. It sets us free of the chains that repress joy and love.

Although you find me often quoting from the New Testament, having been raised as a Jew, I was more often taught to live by the Golden Rule: Do unto others as you would have them do unto you. This covers a wide gamut of situations and I think you will agree, regardless of your own religious persuasion, that the essential message is being taught in every church and temple all over the world. The more we actually put this into practice, the healthier we will be. It is impossible to speak unkindly about someone and love them at the same time. Regarding the Golden Rule, Dr. Reams has said, "Much illness could be prevented, food digestion improved and constipation greatly relieved if more people would live the Golden Rule." He goes on to further say, "So if you want better health, lift up your fellow man."

What we have briefly discussed above is just the beginning of what should become a life-long pursuit of discovering what factors contribute to your illness and which contribute to your health. In a later chapter, we will discuss many often-overlooked factors that can contribute to poor health.

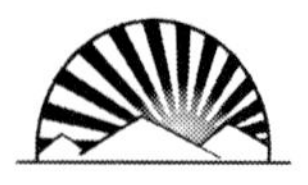

Chapter Three: **How We Heal Naturally**

When one attends a college in the US and learns western medicine, one develops an over-confidence in that system. A lowly medical student becomes almost "brainwashed" to believe that western medicine has just about all the answers and costly research is on the cusp of finding the missing keys to health. Well, I've come a long way since being that lowly medical student and fortunately, I realized early in my career that there were better answers.

No matter what your current burden in life or when you are faced with imminent crisis, the first thing to do is to do nothing except do some deep breathing and pray. I can witness to the fact that God can save you from anything. First, let go and let God.

The reality of faith healing…

I had heard of "faith healers", especially while living in Texas where revival tents were often seen in small towns, but as a Doctor, I scoffed at the notion that God alone could heal an illness.

In 1976 a friend introduced me to a well known "faith healer" who traveled to large cities and staged revivals in civic auditoriums. Just one experience in that setting was enough to convince me that there was a higher healing power than me. I became so fascinated with the healings that took place at my first revival that over the next two years, I would attend many of this same minister's healing revivals in different cities. I saw the crippled walk and the sick made well by the power of faith. How long the results lasted, I did not know but I came to accept that faith in God has healing power.

Within the last two years, Rose had traveled to Florida several times to be with her aging mother the last of which was for her death. Coincidently, we had been watching a revival in Lakeland, Florida over the internet where people were being healed. Rose very much desired to experience this happening and prayed for an opportunity if it was in God's plan. Soon after, she got the call from her brother that the time had come. After her mom's funeral, Rose attended this revival for three days and came away with a renewed personal belief in the power of our Lord.

In July of 2009, we had three women from Florida visit with our church. They were missionaries who were invited to spend time with us in Belize while on their way to Costa Rica. They specialize in spiritual dance and worship. One woman in particular really left Rose with a lasting impression. After our service they engaged in fellowship a while and clicked with each other. She inspired Rose to attend another gathering at the church that evening since another in her party would be speaking. While attending this gathering, Rose was privileged to hear her new found acquaintance also give her personal testimony—she blew Rose away with her story:

From the age of fifteen she developed a crippling form of arthritis. At one point, doctors told her that she would never walk again. It ravaged her whole body. Her childhood sweetheart stuck by her and they eventually married and started a family. Despite difficulties, they had three children—the oldest (a son) later had to help her and care for the youngest. She always refused a wheelchair and had to be carried from place to place. One night, after a painful seventeen years, she prayed with all her heart and soul to Jesus for help and she was shown all the resentments and emotions that she had been harboring for years. She continued in prayer as she had never done before and released a lot of emotions and felt forgiveness for others as well as herself. It was the start of a rebirth of healing that took place over the next nine months after which time she was completely healed and has been serving the Lord ever since. Who would have guessed that she would be involved with spiritual dance? She said that the inspiration came to her when on that prayerful evening she was doing movements in prayer that she had never done before. The Lord then guided her along her path to become a missionary.

Rose later shared with me that she thought this woman was such a powerful light to others of love and joy—a beautiful spirit. She shows no signs of ever have been crippled and she says that she has never detoxed from all the horrific drugs she was taking since childhood...truly a miracle! And to top the story off, Rose had guessed that her age was about forty only to be told that she was age sixty and never even dyed her hair. No special diets or lifestyle changes were then or are now employed—a true testimony to the power of humbling oneself to the Lord. This woman had reached her wits end and brought it all to her Savior. We can never apprehend God's timing. All we can do, in the meantime, is all that we can—continue to act, pray and to be patient.

Our Lord is omnipotent. Pray to Him first in all things. Have faith that God can heal you. I believe that if you do not receive the healing you expect, then you have to make an effort to show God that you “mean business”. I believe that for every step you take towards God, He will take two steps towards you. Whatever your plan, include God as your partner.

Preparation for a natural healing…

Now before you begin, let us evaluate what are your needs? Are you a person in health crisis? If you are, then you have no time to lose in making a 180-degree about-face in your life. If you are not in crisis, then you can make changes more slowly. We will discuss these choices again as they apply.

The following steps are what I advise to regain your health:

- Realize you are the cause and accept blame.
- Decide to take responsibility and make a commitment to change your diet and lifestyle.
- Learn about pH balancing.
- Begin to simplify and purify your diet by eliminating all animal products such as meat, eggs, poultry, fish and dairy.
- Eliminate sugar and all sweeteners.
- Eliminate anything with yeast or that is fermented.
- Purify your drinking water or know your supplier
- Add fresh vegetable juices of carrot and green vegetables to your diet in place of one or more meals
- Learn about colon cleansing options such as self administered enemas
- Learn and plan some intensive cleansing of your body only after thorough education and/or with a trained coach.

The role of Responsibility…

Responsibility is a big word. It is defined in the dictionary as, "involving personal accountability, or being a source or cause". In the previous chapter we discussed why people get sick and you learned that with few exceptions, we are the cause of our illnesses. Now, what are you prepared to do about it?

Accepting responsibility for any phase of our lives takes discipline. It is much easier to lay it off on someone or something else rather than accepting full responsibility. It is much easier to work for someone else than own your own business. It is much easier to eat out rather than cook at home. It is much easier to buy food at the store than raise or grow it yourself. It is much easier to take a package from the freezer to the microwave to your plate than to prepare a meal from all fresh ingredients. It is much easier to consult an "expert" than to self educate. It is much easier to ask a "doctor" to heal us than to invest the time and energy into a process of natural healing.

Let us talk for a moment about another complex word, "perspective". Perspective is the way we view or interpret things. If you were to look at some stationary object in the room where you are now and then move to a different location and view the same object, you would have seen it from two different perspectives.

Our thinking often gets locked into only one point of view on most subjects, when in reality, there is more than one way of viewing most everything. A very wise man is supposed to have said, "There are three sides to every story, your side, my side and the honorable right side." More often than not, we tend to embrace a more commonly accepted "world" view and turn away from the truthful Word of God. Paul urges us in Romans 12:1-2, "…that ye present your bodies a living sacrifice, holy, acceptable unto God, which is your reasonable service. And be not conformed to this world: but be ye transformed by the renewing of your mind, that ye may prove what ***is*** that good, and acceptable, and perfect, will of God."

Accepting personal responsibility for every phase of our lives, not only our health, takes a change in perspective. However, if we accept that we are co-creators with the Lord, we never have to "go it alone". But, taking responsibility usually means change.

If you are ready to take the next step by assuming responsibility for your health, then you are ready to begin to learn how to be healed of illness and how to maintain wellness.

Creating a Personal Plan for Wellness…

Typically, what we find today, are two kinds of approaches to treating illness…

The first and most common approach by most people of the medical profession is to attempt to track down a specific cause of a specific symptom and then to target that with specific drugs, herbs, supplements or whatever is currently suggested as newest and greatest. The second approach, which I favor, is to look at the situation as yes, something is out of balance. Rather than trying to focus narrowly on specific symptoms, let us think of our body as an intricate combination of systems all designed to work together in harmony. This approach requires some inner investigation and acceptance of responsibility for having caused the illness by some imbalance of diet, lifestyle, or thought and, as often is the case, some combination of these.

This is the time to consider your priorities. When we agree to coach a student, we require a minimum three-month commitment to our program. Not that I think or expect all illness to be resolved in three months, but I know that this investment of your time will begin to show you enough results that you will see the benefits of continuing on indefinitely with permanent lifestyle changes. Please make this commitment to your self before beginning our recommended program.

Digestion interferes with the healing process…

We spoke earlier about the miracle of healing that takes place when our body heals itself of a simple skin cut. This built-in, self healing mechanism is but a small example of the miracle of self healing of which our body is capable. In order for the body to heal itself, it needs to use its energy—the same energy that is diverted and spent on digestion—for healing. I can still remember going to grandmas' house for a Thanksgiving dinner. We stuffed ourselves with large portions of a variety of food and then staggered to the couch where we lay like beached whales for the next hour or so, often accompanied by the emission of gas. The digestive process necessary for a large heavy meal takes most of our energy. Gas production after such a meal is a signal of poor digestion.

Aiding digestion is one way of conserving the energy needed for healing. Whenever I go out to a restaurant I often notice that those patrons who received their order well after mine had already completed eating when I was only about halfway done with my own meal. This is because we have become a society that practically inhales their food instead of chewing it thoroughly before swallowing.

Digestion actually begins in the mouth where enzymes begin to break the food down and prepare it for the stomach. The more solid our food is when it reaches the stomach, the more work and enzyme production and energy it takes to break it down further for absorption. The fuel needed for oxidation to take place in each of our tiny cells is not provided by chunks of whatever your last meal was. When eating, keep it in mind that the stomach has no teeth.

Another inhibitor of digestion is the large consumption of liquid people drink to wash down all the un-chewed food. This behavior greatly dilutes the enzymes needed for digestion. Restaurants make a lot of profit on their drinks sold, so it is the first thing that you are asked, "what would you like to drink?" This habit has carried over into our homes too. The best advice that I can give anyone is this: Do not order or have any drinks with their meals—besides, think of all the money that you'll save. Instead, drink at least a half hour before or a half hour after your meal as well as plenty of good water in between.

Now, when you are facing a health crisis, either big or small, we can find good advice written in God's Word. The Bible tells us to fast and pray. Fasting from eating, releases the body to work on healing. However, most people today are too toxic to fast without serious side effects. Poisons that have been stored in various tissues of the body begin to be released during a fast. This is why I strongly advise a carefully planned nutritional program that also rebuilds as well as detoxes together with a very knowledgeable and professional coach. When we fast, the body feeds on unhealthy substances first and when these begin to break down they circulate in the blood. There is also a fine line between fasting and starvation. If we fast long enough or our body has no unhealthy tissue, the body will begin to break down healthy tissue for energy and that is starvation.

The staircase progression of illness...

Earlier I told you that natural healing offers no quick fixes. Western medicine plays upon our fears and attacks symptoms not causes. When your body begins to heal itself at the cellular level and correct vital imbalances often the symptom, like a tumor, may be the last thing to go away. Let me explain further. Picture optimum health as the top step of a flight of stairs and your present illness is at the bottom step. Unless you fell down the flight of stairs and sustained a traumatic injury, you did not suddenly have serious illness. There were progressive symptoms that were ignored on the way down. Look at the following illustration.

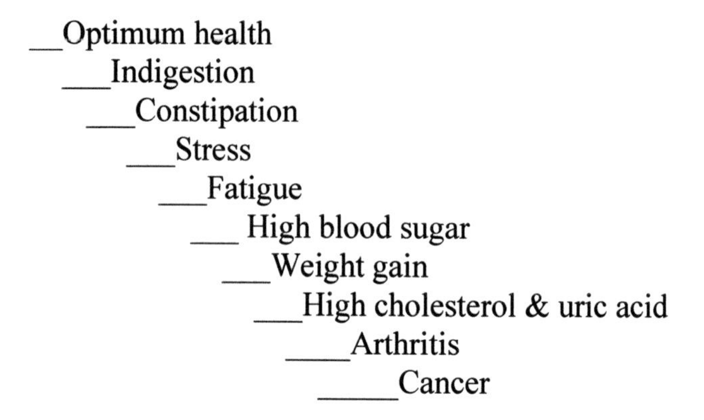

The above illustration shows the slow progression down the flight of stairs from optimum health to serious illness—this is how the body regresses. The process slowly happens in reverse as various imbalances are corrected.

Toxicity builds up over time...

Well, to begin with, it is often said that a picture is worth a thousand words. So, please try to visualize that a reasonably well kept home typically has a waste basket in every room. When filled to capacity (or before) they would have to be emptied or "stuff" would start to over flow onto the floor and then would probably begin to get kicked around the house if something wasn't done about it, right? Eventually, the home would be filled with all kinds of debris and would soon become too unsanitary and unsafe to live in. It is also scientifically said that each person has between seventy and one-hundred trillion cells in their body that also serve as receptacles (just like those waste baskets). All the toxins, over the years, that we ingest, inhale or absorb through our skin are not getting eliminated as you might like to think. They are being stored in these trillions of cells which actually have the more important work of maintaining healthy functioning of our body.

So, what happens when our cells are overloaded with toxins and the accumulated waste products of our metabolism—the process of converting the nutrients from the food we eat into energy? These begin to overload the entire system.

Particular organs of our body have the task of disposing of these toxins. These include the liver, spleen, kidneys, lungs, skin, several of the mucus membranes and the colon. Our blood is a major highway, both for delivery of digested food to each cell and for the removal of the cells waste products to the organs of detoxification. However, try to picture what happens if each of these vital organs is overloaded with "garbage". The result is the blood can not release its' load nor can it accept any more from each of the cells. Thus, we have a serious backlog of toxic waste interfering with normal body function and our body—just like our house—will soon become unhealthy. How will it become unhealthy? Each of us will have different symptoms from "colds", allergies, arthritis, diabetes, to cancer etc.

Intensive Cleansing

From many years of experience, I believe that the best way to detoxify and heal the body is by learning the skills of a seven-day intensive cleanse. This includes the entire alimentary canal of your body going from your mouth to your rectum.

Why Do We Do a Seven-Day Intensive Cleanse?

Our modified intensive cleansing program is a synergistic combination of the essence of proven modern and ancient techniques. I believe that there is something special about a seven-day cleanse. "Seven" is considered by many as the number of deity, such as the seven day creation etc. Many researchers believe that the body attempts to replace every cell every seven years. In regard to intestinal and tissue cleansing, we have found that many more beneficial results occur from the fourth to the seventh day of an intensive program, than occur on the first to the third days. Mucous linings in our intestinal tract need to be eliminated before the encrusted old fecal matter lodged in the folds and kinks can be loosened and flushed out. These pockets of putrefaction are the beginnings of polyps, cancer, multiple disease entities and finally death. This thickened wall prevents our body from absorbing the nutrition it needs to be healthy and the build up of harmful toxins leak into our blood stream. Thus, our immune system is compromised. From my many years of experience, I know that it takes several seven-day intensive cleanses to begin to eliminate years of buildup. (See Appendices A-H complete details)

What Happens After the Seven Days?

In between each of the recommended Seven-Day Cleanses attention is paid to maintaining and improving the body's

pH chemistry, eliminating parasites and Candida (yeast). Intensive detoxification of the colon will remove the "good" as well as the unwanted "bad" bacteria inside of our body, thus, we balance our program with the replacement of "good" bacteria as well. All of these factors must be addressed and play a critical role in diminishing our body's ability to heal itself. A healthy immune system is a strong defense.

Get the Supportive Coaching You Need…

Generally speaking, I recommend a series of Seven-Day Cleansing programs with breaks in between because this is what was taught to me and it works—why mess with success? Each student that we work with will have unique requirements and circumstances and I pay close attention to what they and their body results are telling me. Together we determine what may work best for that individual due to physical and/or time restraints.

If you want to go this on your own that is okay too, provided that you are well disciplined at following advice and instructions to the "T" and do not try to over exert yourself or deprive yourself nutritionally. Intensive cleansing is not for the novice to attempt without careful study and supervision. Toxins may be dumped too rapidly causing toxemia. Very careful dietary plans must be adhered to in order to maintain energy levels which are essential for healing to occur. The proven procedures and training schedules we teach are designed to prevent complications plus our personal coaching keeps you on top of every situation that may occur. When questions arise, have someone you know with experience in cleansing be available to you. Let them know beforehand what you are planning and most importantly, have friends and family members offer to be supportive of your goals and accomplishments.

Dietary Considerations…

After thirty years of research, teaching and investigating many different dietary considerations, it seems clear that some form of a "cleansing diet" is essential not only during detoxification, but also for periodic rejuvenation as well. What sort of "cleansing diet" produces the best result may vary because of different parameters?

Example 1: Individual who is very toxic and in life threatening condition-

Drastic Measures must be initiated immediately.

Example 2: An Individual subject to chronic illness
Example 3: An Individual with an acute illness
Example 4: An individual wishing to delay aging

Each of the above examples, when combined with considerations of lifestyle and motivation, will necessitate different dietary/nutritional regimens. However, all the above being said, I like to teach a basic cleansing diet of the following regimen:

Basic Cleansing Diet

NO Tea, coffee (except enemas), soft drinks or anything carbonated, no sweeteners except pure maple syrup (sparingly), no dairy, no eggs, cheese, breads of any kind, no grains except specified, no meat or fish, no micro-waved foods, salt, black pepper, no pickles or prepared foods, margarines, smoked or processed foods.

YES Fresh or steamed/stir-fry vegetables; Fresh or steamed fruit; Baked potato; Steamed rice or millet once daily; Cooked beans or almonds daily; Garlic and onions; Fresh vegetable juices and other "live foods"; fresh green coconut water; Herbal teas; *pure water—½ body weight in ounces Daily Minimum—and extra virgin olive oil.

In addition, it seems evident that a diet that is mostly alkaline helps the body to heal itself and then keeping the body slightly alkaline promotes wellness. Most biochemists who are natural healing orientated recommend the following parameters:

Alkaline Food Intake – 75% - 80% Daily
Acidic Food Intake – 20% - 25% Daily
Complex Carbohydrates – 80% Daily
Proteins – 15% Daily
Fats – 5% Daily

Other cleansing diets are sometimes more specific to certain conditions and individual criteria and they are taught on an individual basis.

Whether you feel good or really terrible...

Last, but not least, a Seven-Day Cleanse can benefit everyone. This program is not just for the seriously ill. Why wait until you really become sick? No matter how healthy you think you are, you can only get better. My wife and I make a point of doing a "maintenance-cleanse" at least once or twice a year. For those of you who are suffering, it works best to begin this program before your body has already been compromised by drugs, radiation or surgery. But, if you feel that you have no where else to turn after "modern" medicine hasn't worked for you, then I am inclined to say that there is still hope if you can approach this program with vigor and the determination to be well again.

In my opinion, nothing eliminates toxins and rebuilds the body without doing harm like intensive tissue/organ cleansing. This regimen requires complete devotion to healing yourself, maintaining your health, and gradually learning how to adapt to a new lifestyle.

At the present time, we offer a cleansing program with coaching via our web site: naturalcleansingtechniques.com. We require a ninety-day commitment to our program because we know that it takes a minimum of three months to begin to undo many years of neglect. In my opinion, most health problems can be undeniably improved in ninety days with a combination of intensive cleansing and other natural healing techniques that work synergistically to heal and not harm. A sound maintenance program with periodic intensive and other targeted cleanses will insure health by eliminating and preventing the building up of toxins.

The optimum schedule for the intensive cleansing program is:

1. Seven-Day Intensive Cleansing Program
2. Seven-Day Maintenance Program
3. Seven-Day Intensive Cleansing Program
4. 10 day Parasite program plus maintenance
5. Seven-Day Intensive Cleansing Program
6. 10-day Parasite program plus maintenance

To insure greater success and to avoid any distress on your physical body we strongly recommend that you start with a Basic Cleansing Diet for several days before a Seven-Day Intensive if you have been eating an animal based diet. It is also advisable to begin honing your skill at giving yourself an enema. (See Appendix B: Instructions for taking an Enema)

Cleansing the Colon with Enemas…

Initially, most everyone seems to be turned off to the concept of enemas. I remember all too vividly when I was a very young child and taken to the pediatricians office and was pronounced to have had some kind of intestinal virus for which special enemas were prescribed. My mother administered the first one to me and not only was I mortified but also I couldn't stand the pressure of fluid in my lower bowel. I don't remember more than one attempt.

When first presented with the regimen for detoxification by Dr. William Donald Kelley, I was aghast at the prospect of administering an enema to myself of any kind, much less the type that Dr. Kelley recommended. Now, having been informed of the purpose, function, and proper procedure of taking an enema, I began to relax and to enjoy its many benefits. It relieves distress, increases a sense of well-being and cleanliness by removing toxins and debris from the colon which is essential in all conditions of ill health and especially if you have cancer.

This is not the same as having someone else quickly force some liquid into you—not at all. Remember, you are in control and you will tune in to what is going on in your body at all times. Getting oneself comfortable with self-administration of enemas will take some mental and physical practice. If you are a novice, I recommend beginning with one of the Fleet Brand pre-packaged enema kits available at most drug stores/pharmacies. Then progress to purchasing a two-quart combination douche/enema bag. This should be the fountain style with the open top, or preferably an enema canister (see Appendix A: Instructions for Making an Enema Canister) that can be cleaned easily. After you feel proficient at dealing with a one-quart warm water enema you are ready to graduate to a more advanced colon cleansing.

Be sure to block off 1–1½ hours for taking your enema with quiet and no interruptions! When you have your own routine down, it will take you less time but do not rush Mother Nature.

Why a coffee enema, you ask? The best explanation of all that I have read is one explained by Max Gerson, MD in his classic book, *A Cancer Therapy*. Dr. Gerson states that, "Patients have to know that coffee enemas are not given for the function of the intestines but for the stimulation of the liver." He goes on to explain that the result is an increased production of bile caused by the coffee producing a peristalsis at the hepatic flexure where the hepatic duct empties bile into the colon. Dr. Kelley advised using a colon tube to assure that the fluid of the enema reaches the ascending colon where many problems originate (see illus. VI-c on pg.44). The hepatic flexure is at the top of the ascending colon and the appendix is at the bottom where debris often gets backed up and causes inflammation hence "appendicitis".

I must interject here and mention that the removal of the appendix eliminates our God given warning signal that something is terribly amiss in our colon that will lead to more serious illness if not corrected. We must treat the cause and not the symptom. Once the appendix is removed, the problem is now "out of sight and out of mind" until the next serious symptom occurs. Too often, the early warning signs are ignored until you or your doctor feels that there is no other option but surgery. Once successfully performed, never assume that you or a loved one is completely out of the woods. This is the time for some serious colon cleansing, diet and lifestyle change in order to renew and maintain the health of your body.

Returning to the topic of coffee enemas, a colon tube is not absolutely essential. Dr. Gerson was advocating coffee enemas without one but I think they aid in producing better results. Another important consideration is the replacement of "good" bacteria when colon cleansing. Supplements can be oral or rectal implants.

Every enema will be different for you. Sometimes all goes smoothly, most of the time not so smoothly. Don't be discouraged. Learn to enjoy the quiet, meditative experience you can create by getting into this very powerful self-administered, body cleansing tool—detailed in Appendix B. Other types of enemas can also be very helpful and should be studied. As additional study, I recommend *Tissue Cleansing through Bowel Management* by Dr. Bernard Jenson; *Death Begins in the Colon* by V.E. Irons; and *A Cancer Therapy* by Max Gerson, MD.

Colon cleansing is an essential skill to learn for improved health. When someone becomes ill it is usually the result of a gradual decline in wellness not detected early enough or ignored. Wellness is a lifestyle and we must learn to tune-in to our inner self and thus be able to make small mini-course corrections rather than waiting until a health crisis forces us to more drastic methods. Natural healing does not produce an immediate reversal of illness, but a slow retreating back up the path of decline. Along the way, "healing crises" will occur which means that temporary exacerbations of previous illnesses not completely resolved are taking place. These exacerbation changes are usually considered a positive change and are dealt with by more frequent colon cleanses.

Regarding Supplements...

We advocate a basic cleansing/detoxification program as the way to begin healing for everyone. Then, depending on the results, more specific supplements and/or regimens may be advised. However, I will make a generalized statement that in my opinion minerals are much more important than vitamins. Once again, I will say that most illness occurs from the lack of the proper minerals.

As I am writing this book, we are actively teaching quite a few people including a lady in residence who was diagnosed with metastatic breast cancer, which recent x-ray revealed has spread into her bones. A friend and former student came to visit her and she was surprised that the same basic program, with some minor changes, was being taught for the cancer as we had taught her for another health problem. "What about using herbs to kill the cancer, she asked?" "Well," I said, "if you know of some herbs that will kill cancer please let me know." And, I said, "You have forgotten your lessons that whether it is a cold or a cancer, with few exceptions, we bring illness upon ourselves. The body is out of balance. If, after cleansing the body, health does not begin to return, then it is time to look at adding something else to the basic regimen."

It has been my observation that most natural health care professionals have substituted food supplements like herbs, vitamins and remedies for the prescription drugs used by conventional medicine. They practice "shot-gun therapy." This means that by shooting a wide pattern of lots of ammunition, you have got to hit something. Your local health food store will gladly load you up with a multitude of the latest and greatest in the hope that something will work to alleviate your symptoms. Or you may have already tried a multitude of supplements that you have heard of or read about. You are a willing participant in this method because you are also convinced that there must be some herb or vitamin available that will make you well without your having to change anything about your lifestyle which caused the illness.

Usually, when we interview a prospective new student for our cleansing program, they want to show us all the supplements they have been taking presently or in the past. My first question is, “If all those things worked for you, then why did you come to us?”

On the contrary, we believe in taking as few supplements as possible and using high quality food as our medicine after detoxifying and rebuilding. Our wish is to eventually take no supplements because we produce most of our own food and live a healthy lifestyle. More will be discussed about this in our chapter on diet.

Once again I want to assure you that we have no financial interest in any product discussed in this book. It is my goal to reduce our need for supplements and invest the money into better quality food. However, in order to do a thorough cleansing and rebuilding of the body special supplements and some supplies are needed, more initially and less as healing occurs. The supplements and supplies that we currently advise you to purchase have been carefully chosen for quality, value and usefulness. It is very possible, however, that by the time you read this book, we may have tweaked our recommended supplements a little. Let me proceed to explain the rationale for each item listed in Appendix C:

1. **Minerals**: We have used Min-Col for many years. It is calcium plus trace minerals. It was developed by Dr. Reams and is quality controlled.
2. **Magnesium Oxide powder**, NOW brand, to balance calcium
3. **Food Grade Diatomaceous Earth** (fossil shell flour): Composed of 84% Silicon Dioxide (Silica), the benefits are numerous and can be found online at: www.EarthWorksHealth.com. Silica plays an important role in many body functions and has a direct relationship to mineral absorption
4. **Rutin**, which comes from buckwheat, helps maintain the health of small blood vessels many of which are found in our brain. In some instances we advise using this in combination with vitamin C.
5. **Willow** is the plant from which aspirin was synthesized. It is a natural anti-inflammatory and may slightly act as a blood thinner and should be discontinued before surgery.
6. **Capsicum** or cayenne from red pepper is one of the most healthful herbs. It helps to normalize blood pressure, improves circulation and digestion.
7. **Probiotics**: Beneficial bacteria, to offset Candida, (yeast) comes in many forms. We particularly like Yeast Away from Peak Health Care because it not only contains good bacteria but also an enzyme to break down the cell wall of the yeast.
8. **Oregano Oil**: Of all the brands we try, we still think that Oreganol is the best. We advise using it internally to combat viruses and infections (instead of antibiotics) and externally on infected bites and sores. Internally it will also kill good bacteria like antibiotics and should be used discreetly with probiotic replacement.
9. **Tea Tree Oil** is an excellent topical for bites, infections, and fungus.

10. **Pancreatin**: I consider pancreatic enzymes to be of primary importance when doing an intestinal cleansing program. They help to break down mucous linings in the bowel; help to break down un-digested protein; and help to dissolve the protein shell wall of tumors. However not all pancreatic enzymes are the same. In my opinion the most important component of a pancreatic enzyme should be chymotripsin. This is not found in enzymes of plant origin but only in animal pancreas gland and although I do not advise eating swine, the pancreatin from pigs seems to produce the best result because pigs are the animal most like humans. NOW brand Pancreatin fills this requirement at the best price we have found thus far.
11. **Kelp** provides sea minerals, iron and iodine for the liver and thyroid. Algazim is Norwegian kelp, a quality product at a fair price.
12. **Green food** supplement for energy boost should not be mostly algae or spirulina as most are, but contain mainly dried grasses and grains.
13. **Bentonite clay** helps to draw out toxins and radiation from the bowel when combined with psyllium as a bulking agent. We particularly like Pascalite brand which seems to make a smoother drink than some others.
14. **Psyllium** can be ground whole or husks but buy plain not mixed with anything—such as added herbs.
15. **Flax seed**, organic if possible, is used for making a drink from the extracted oil which contains essential fatty acids.
16. **Extra Virgin Olive Oil** is an excellent source of amino acids and vitamin E and it is used for liver and gallbladder cleansing.
17. **Epsom salts** is sometimes used for an oral flushing of the digestive tract

18. **Light roast organic coffee** is used for enemas and can be obtained from www.sawilsons.com .
19. **Para-Cleanse** from Nature's Sunshine is a quality product.
20. **Test paper** for urine/saliva pH can be obtained from Pike Labs in Strong, ME.
21. **Luffa** for dry skin brushing
22. The best **juicer** is the Norwalk; the next best is the Green Star: The Norwalk is the "Rolls Royce" of juicers. It has a shredder and a hydraulic press both built into the same unit and produces juice with no friction or heat meaning more fresh enzymes and highest quality juice. Our latest cost check was $2,500.US. The Green Star is a high quality heavy duty juice extractor similar outwardly to a Champion, but the motor drives twin stainless steel gears which slowly spin towards each other crushing the fruit or vegetable with little heat then strained into a pitcher. Our latest cost check was about $500 US.
23. **Enema bag or canister** needs to hold 2 quarts of liquid. A fountain syringe douche style bag is best or a canister. A canister can be home-made by purchasing a 2-qt. plastic juice container with a lid, a coned shaped brass fitting used for a air hose or LP gas hose, about 3ft. of 5/16" (outer) X ¼" (inner) clear plastic tubing and a tip and clamp from an old enema bag.
24. **Colon catheters** are becoming hard to get and expensive. We like a 30" 28fr red rubber by Bard. A catheter assures that enema fluid gets into the ascending colon.
25. **"Big Berkey"** is an exceptional counter-top, gravity flow water purifier.

Moving right along...

Let me not bog you down at this time with detailed instructions for completing a 90-day program of total body cleansing. We have provided you with all this information in the appendices in the back of this book. Since I have discussed the benefits of cleaning the colon, let us now consider other areas of the body and how to cleanse them and why…

Cleansing Other Organs of Detoxification

The Liver is a major organ of detoxification...

As a major organ of detoxification, I am putting it mildly when I say that the liver has a lot to handle. In today's society where convenience and self-indulgence is the order of the day, we contaminate ourselves on a regular basis with chemical pollutants, environmental pollutants, food preservatives and additives such as color, emulsifiers, stabilizers, and sweeteners. You can then add alcoholic and carbonated beverages, deodorants, hairsprays, and the list goes on and on. All of these things, along with your body's metabolic wastes are to be removed by the liver. Excessive stress on our liver causes damage to the liver and a damaged liver, say from hepatitis, cirrhosis of the liver, infectious mononucleosis or other damage, reduces its ability to handle toxicity. So, this vital organ needs to be respected (same as the rest of our body) and not abused if we want to maintain a healthy body. However, the Liver is the only organ that can re-generate itself, to my knowledge and so there is hope.

Flushing the gallbladder and liver...

One procedure that helps keep the liver as well as the colon clean is the coffee enema that I discussed earlier in this chapter. For now, I would like to emphasize that one of the most important procedures for persons over twenty-five years of age is the liver/gallbladder flush. This helps to release accumulated fats and toxins stored in the fat of these organs. We recommend this procedure to our students usually after the first or second week of intensive cleansing and then repeated every six months. If you are not already on a cleansing program or special diet, then I suggest first going on a restrictive diet for a few days or if need be, even longer. Do this by eliminating all animal products, fats and sugar, as well, if you want to get good results. At the same time, by incorporating coffee enemas into your daily routine you could probably forego the Epsom salts which aide in evacuation.

The steps in doing this are not difficult and are as follows:

1. From Monday through Saturday noon, you should drink as much lemon, lime or white grapefruit juice, as your appetite will permit (preferably organic), in addition to regular meals. You may use frozen or bottled juice (I am very leery of bottled juices) purchased from the health food store or the supermarket only if juice made from fresh fruit is not available. Be sure to read the labels and obtain a type of juice that has no additives whatsoever. Also be sure to eat only a vegetarian or cleansing diet, no food of animal origin.
2. At noon on Saturday, eat a vegetarian lunch.
3. Three hours later, take two teaspoons of "Epsom Salts" dissolved in about one cup of hot water. If the taste is objectionable it may be followed by a little citrus juice, (freshly squeezed if possible).
4. Two hours later, repeat the "Epsom Salts".
5. For the evening meal, you may have a grapefruit, grapefruit juice, lemon or lime juice or fresh vegetable juice.

6. At bedtime, you have two choices:
   - Take one half (1/2) cup of warm *unrefined olive oil followed by a Small glass (1/2 cup or more) of grapefruit, lemon or lime juice, or
   - Take one half (1/2) cup of warm *unrefined olive oil blended with one half (1/2) cup of citrus juice.

*Unrefined, extra virgin, cold pressed olive oil can be purchased from your health food store (buy only in cans or light proof glass; no plastic).

7. Go immediately to bed and lie on your right side with the right knee pulled up close to the chest for thirty minutes.

8. The next morning, one hour before breakfast, repeat the "Epsom Salts"

Continue your cleansing diet or nutritional program.

If the "Epsom Salts" proves too harsh at any time, then substitute warm/hot water and lime/lemon/grapefruit juice.

Most persons have reported slight to moderate nausea when taking the olive oil-citrus juice, which slowly disappears by the time you go to sleep. Should you vomit the olive oil, it need not be repeated at this time. Chances are that you aren't going to vomit—only very rarely does this ever happen. This flushing of the liver and gall bladder (if present) stimulates and cleans the liver as no other system does.

Oftentimes, persons suffering from gallstones, billowiness, backaches, nausea, etc. for years find gall stone type objects in the stool the following day. These objects are light green to dark green in color, very irregular in shape, gelatinous in texture, and vary in size from "grape seeds" to "cherries". If there seems to be a large number of these objects in the stool, the liver flush should be repeated in two weeks.

Cleansing the kidneys...

The kidneys filter approximately 4,000 quarts of blood daily—another amazing feat that we totally take for granted. The wastes, largely urea, are eliminated and the acid/alkaline balance is maintained—an extremely important factor that I discuss in the chapter on diet. This is facilitated by the drinking of plenty of liquids taken daily. It goes without saying, we must drink beneficial liquids—free of toxins—otherwise we impede this natural process. Now, some high volume soda drinkers may be saying, “but I drink lots of liquid doesn’t that replace some of the required water?” Although soda manufacturers start out with purified water, their end result becomes toxic to the body due to the added chemicals such as colorants, preservatives, flavoring agents, caffeine, as well as large quantities of sugar or artificial sweetener and the metabolic waste product of carbon dioxide. Have I said enough?

Healthy individuals eating a well-balanced diet with plenty of vegetables and some fruit should drink pure spring water, or purified water (know your source). You may however, substitute with the juice of vegetables and fruits, preferably made fresh (without other additives or sugar) or fresh green coconut water which has other added benefits. Drinking fresh vegetable juices will help to supplement a poor diet. If juices are being consumed more freely, it is better to get into the habit of diluting them with fresh water in order to minimize the amount of natural sugar in your diet. Consuming enough water throughout the day is essential. A rule to consider is to consume ½ your body weight in ounces of water daily. Therefore a 150-pound person needs to consume at least 75 ounces of water daily spread over the day in addition to other liquids—critical in balancing and maintaining your body chemistry.

Cleansing the lungs...

Anyone reading this book knows that our lungs are for breathing. So, the focus of this discussion is first on the importance of proper breathing—life is dependent upon the adequate exchanges of gases in the lungs. The most significant is the removal of carbon dioxide and the flow of oxygen into the blood. Most of us do not think twice about our pattern of breathing because it is automatic, right? Well, yes, unconsciously we all continue to breathe due to our autonomic nervous system but to what extent do we truly give ourselves what our bodies need for optimum health?

Except for diseases associated with smoking, the respiratory organs have been largely ignored. By understanding a few basic principles of how the respiratory process operates and interacts with the body and mind, we can gain deeper insight as to how our body functions on many other levels. The effects of breathing extend far beyond the physical transfer of air in and out of the body—they extend to the workings of the heart and lungs as well as to subtle molecular processes through which the body's energy production is maintained.

All life forms are composed of tiny living units called cells, each requiring a continuous source of energy. Our body's tissues and organs are composed of these cells and they must function properly in order to keep us alive. The nutrients supplied by the food we eat act as a fuel but it must be converted into a form that these individual cells can use or we would die.

Breathing effects energy supply...

Energy is produced through a process of combustion when oxygen combines with a fuel. A typical example of this is when we build a camp fire which produces carbon dioxide, water, heat and light. Naturally, a rapidly burning system such as this could not take place within our bodies and still keep us alive. However, when fuel is burned at an exceptionally slow rate there is no visible light and a steady source of energy is maintained. This process takes place in tiny subunits within the cell called mitochondria. These contain a series of specialized protein molecules or enzymes which transfer the energy released from the oxidation of our food to a storage molecule called adenosine triphosphate, or ATP. ATP has the ability to deliver energy within the cells of the body—this energy, in turn, maintains the chemical reactions necessary for the cells to function normally.

Thus, the process of respiration occurs within the cell where nutrient fuel is burned with oxygen to release energy. The nose, trachea (windpipe), lungs, circulatory system, and attending muscles all act to transport oxygen from the air we breathe to make it readily available to individual cells. Each of these organs plays a crucial role in determining oxygen supply, and therefore the amount of energy available to cells throughout the body. Energy production within the body could potentially be altered should any of these involved organs not function properly. It stands to reason that an insufficient supply of oxygen to meet the body's energy demands would result in a reduction of cellular function or even death.

Breathing patterns can take a toll...

This leads us to a little recognized fact, that the importance of maintaining health is directly related to the quality of our breathing.

When we pay attention, we see that breathing is diaphragmatic or thoracic, continuous or interrupted by pauses, rhythmical or irregular—all affected by either our physical or emotional state. We have all experienced changes in our breathing under varying circumstances such as fear, anger, sorrow and physical exertion—so each event affects the breath. The opposite is also true. If we intentionally or unconsciously alter our pattern of breathing, it will affect our physical and emotional state. Some of us have unintentionally set up physical responses to emotional triggers that over time become a habitual pattern of behavior. In other words, we interrupt a natural and healthy process of breathing. To correct the ill effects of this upon our mind and body we need to pay attention to these patterns and practice quality breathing.

With repeated efforts, over time, we can re-train our muscles and automatic responses through breathing exercises to have a direct influence on our body's total health.

There is much more that can be said about the process of breathing than is said here. This page is intended as a basic introduction to the principle that quality breathing is essential to good health. I encourage each and every one of you to pay more attention to your breathing.

We need to learn and incorporate deep breathing into our regular breathing pattern. Deep breathing should really be called, and often is, diaphragmatic breathing because the use of the diaphragm is critical. The diaphragm I am talking about is the large muscular structure above your stomach and under your lungs, not a birth control device.

Place the palm of either hand just above your stomach. Now slowly inhale through your nose as you push out your lower chest against your hand. Fill your lungs and now slowly exhale through your mouth and feel your abdomen contracting. Try it again. Once you get the idea you are ready to graduate to the next level. Inhale slowly as before but count slowly to six as you fill your lungs completely. Hold this breath to the count of three and now slowly exhale through your mouth to the count of six again emptying your lungs. Hold this for another three-count and begin the next inhale etc.

If you have never practiced deep breathing in this manner it will undoubtedly feel awkward at first. The more you practice it when walking or bouncing on a rebounder—or anytime you consciously think of it—not only will it become more comfortable, but, believe it or not, it can become automatic without conscious thought. Practicing enough during your waking hours will eventually allow you to breathe more deeply when you sleep.

Why a nasal wash?

The nasal passages are lined with a thin layer of mucus that is one of our body's first lines of defense against disease. Many impurities are also given off by the lungs, thus helping to detoxify the body. Some of these same impurities get trapped in the mucus lining of the nose. Actually, they can hardly be avoided since most every environment in which we breathe contains impurities that we also inhale. A nasal wash keeps this layer of mucus moist, clean and healthy. This can be incorporated into your daily routine.

The simple routine of irrigating the nose each morning is often overlooked. You can accomplish this by sniffing water into the nose and then blowing it out. This should be repeated several times. Once the nose is cleansed, deep breathing can take place. One should breathe as deeply as possible in the fresh air for about twelve minutes a day as a healthy practice.

An alternative method of nasal irrigation that I also recommend is frequent rinsing using a saline solution of warm salty water with the aide of a sinus irrigation system or what is otherwise known as a nasal irrigation pot and follow the easy instructions that are supplied with it. However, a bulb syringe will work also. Most packaged nasal irrigation systems sold in stores utilize a saline solution. You can make your own home-made saline solution by dissolving a combination of ¼ teaspoon of real sea salt and 1/8 teaspoon of baking soda (optional) per one cup of purified water.

Use it anytime to:

- Remove excess mucus due to congestion.
- Relieve congestion from swollen linings of the nose and sinuses
- Rid nostrils of pollen and other allergens.
- Cleanse the nasal membranes of airborne contaminants, such as dust or smoke.
- Relieve nasal dryness due to air travel, air conditioning or climate conditions.
- Reduce infection by rinsing with an anti-viral or anti-fungal solution

- Improve flow of breath before doing relaxation or meditation techniques.

Here's what to do:

1. Put your head over the sink and tilt your head to one side with one nostril over the other one.
2. Squirt the bulb syringe into the upper nostril. The solution should run from the upper nostril up into your sinus cavity and through and out your lower nostril.
3. Gently blow excess mucus from your nose.
4. Repeat steps 1-3 for the other nostril.

Cleaning the skin...

Most people overlook the fact that the skin is an organ. Everyone desires to have attractive clear healthy looking skin and yet few consider it as an important organ of detoxification. When large amounts of poisons accumulate in the body, all systems are overloaded and this function of the skin comes into play. As a result, all kinds of eruptions, odors, colors, and blemishes will appear on the skin. Instead of just trying to cover it up and apply product on the surface of the skin, we need to eliminate the cause of the problem on the inside of our body. These conditions will disappear as the body becomes detoxified.

Personally, I prefer to take a comfortably cool shower each day or as needed, using castile soap or a good natural soap such as Dr. Bronner's, which can be purchased from the health food store. Try to avoid ingesting or immersing your body in water chemically treated with fluoride and chlorine (a man-made inorganic form of chlorine) by installing a filtering shower head if necessary. Hot showers can be especially unhealthy when using chlorinated water since the heat will open the pores of your skin and you will absorb more chemicals. Don't neglect shampooing your hair regularly. After your shower or bath, the skin should be rubbed briskly with a towel or "Luffa"—a dry fibrous sponge from the fruit of a plant— until a warm glow is felt.

What are the benefits of dry skin brushing?

Dry skin brushing is an excellent practice to be done before showering and primarily serves to exfoliate the skin by the removal of dead skin cells. This helps improve skin texture and cell renewal—a good thing for those people who are concerned with appearances. More importantly, however, this practice opens up the pores and allows the skin to breathe. Skin brushing plays a significant role in detoxification of the body. Here are some interesting facts:

- The Skin is the largest organ of the body.
- The Skin is responsible for 25% of the body's daily detoxification.
- The Skin eliminates 2lbs. of waste acids daily.
- The Skin receives $^1/_3$ of all the blood circulating in the body.
- The Skin will reveal problems related to blood toxicity.
- The Skin is the last to receive nutrients in the body while the first to show signs of imbalance or deficiency.

Since dry skin brushing increases the circulation to the skin, it encourages your body's natural discharge of wastes especially aiding drainage of your lymphatic system whose job it is to remove toxins from the blood and other vital tissues. By eliminating clogged pores, dry skin brushing helps your skin to absorb nutrients while also aiding in proper excretion of metabolic wastes. Furthermore, nerve endings in the skin also become stimulated and help to rejuvenate your nervous system. So, the benefits of dry skin brushing are more than just skin deep.

Dry skin brushing is a perfect addition to a healthy regimen for all natural health enthusiasts and I recommend this practice to all my students. The cosmetic industry has made natural bristle brushes for this purpose readily available in health stores and drug stores, etc

What is the best way to practice dry skin brushing?

You should only use a loofa (or Luffa) sponge or a natural bristle brush, preferably one with a long handle and a detachable head with a hand strap. This will enable you to comfortably reach and work all areas of your body.

Get into the habit of brushing once a day prior to your bath or shower while your skin is dry and unclothed. Always brush towards your heart starting with your feet first working upward and then from your hands towards your shoulders with long sweeping strokes. Move onto your torso while continuing to overlap your brush strokes several times in each area in the direction of your heart. Skip over any broken or sensitive areas of your skin.

After dry brushing, you can further invigorate your skin and stimulate circulation by alternating hot and cold temperatures of water while rinsing in the shower. Add to this, towel drying yourself vigorously and you have completed your daily regimen.

Keep your brush clean and free of mildew by washing it with soapy water at least once a week and allowing it to dry thoroughly after rinsing in an airy, well lit area, preferably in the sun.

Persistence is the key to this program—only over a prolonged period of about a month will you experience its full benefits. I also highly suggest, as with any detoxification program, that if you are feeling ill, you can rid yourself of more toxins quicker by repeating this regimen twice a day, as well as increasing the number of coffee enemas you are taking.

A true healing and wellness program takes time and effort. Remember that you did not get the way you are overnight.

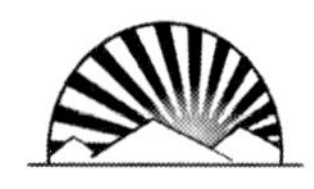

Chapter Four: **What Is A Healthy Diet?**

People are more addicted to their foods than drug addicts are to the most dangerous drugs. Changing someone's diet from unhealthy to healthy is a major challenge. "What we can conceive, we can achieve." This wise quotation sums up the essence of any situation. First, we have to educate ourselves to understand why dietary or any change is necessary. Once we grasp the concept, then the mind can lead the body in the right direction. What is the best diet? This question has been asked time and again over centuries. My belief is that a vegetarian diet is the healthiest diet—see, if you will, if my reasoning resonates with you also.

There are numerous translations of the Bible and other historical documents. Their accuracy depends on the particular understanding and philosophy of those doing the translating. Words are oftentimes translated and taken for their literal meaning—conforming to the simplest and most obvious and commonly understood use—rather than acknowledging that their derivation or use at a particular time in history was different. For instance, the word "meat" is found nineteen times in the New Testament and it would appear as though Jesus sanctioned the eating of meat. However, the Greek word that is translated into the English word "meat" should more accurately be translated to mean "food" or "nourishment". If you can accept this viewpoint, then I think you will be more open to the idea that vegetarianism is the healthier diet.

Similar mistranslations have possibly occurred with the use of the word “fish”. According to some scholars, the Greek word for the word “fish”, namely “Ichthus”, translates as Jesus Christ Son of God Savior. Apparently, in the early church, the word fish was used as a secret term and the fish is still symbolically used today. Since Jesus taught in metaphors and parables, it is conceivable that its use in the New Testament was used to convey the deeper meaning of the feeding of the higher teachings of God rather than the eating of dead fish. Others have also pointed out that during that era and Babylonian times, a submarine plant called the fish plant was used for food, and the word plant could have been lost in the translation. In any case, due to different historical accounts and the translations of what few documented writings remain, the question of whether or not Jesus was a vegetarian is a delicate subject and very highly debated. Certainly, after conducting ones own thorough investigation this is a personal decision for each of us to make.

The Dead Sea Scrolls indirectly suggest that Jesus was a vegetarian because they point to His relationship with the Essenes. Jesus and His parents were Nazarenes who were thought of as having been part of this unique group of Jews. The Essenes required a discipline and purity of mind, body and spirit that went beyond the common day practice of other Jews of the time. Several hundred years before the coming of Jesus they adhered to the highest meaning of the Law of Moses which said “Thou shalt not kill.” This meant absolutely no consumption of meat or the killing of animals not even for sacrifice. Their focus was primarily on God and so they set themselves apart in the peace of the desert where they developed self-sufficient communities. According to historical documents other than the Bible, Jesus escaped to an Essene community in order to avoid being killed by King Herod. It was there that He was raised and trained in a teaching that taught compassion and love for all life including animals. Thus, Jesus began His life as a vegetarian and despite arguments to the contrary, I believe that He lived out His entire life as a vegetarian.

There are many sound and moral arguments for vegetarianism today—such as non-cruelty to animals, preserving the Earth, and eliminating world hunger and starvation, just by redirecting water, land and energy resources being spent on a meat-centered diet. However, our primary concern here is the enormous benefit to our health. We have come to be so far removed from our basic and wholesome beginnings...

If we go back in time before the coming of Jesus, the Old Testament of the Bible talks about the Garden of Eden where Adam and Eve were first introduced to eating in an environment that was ideal and eternal. Genesis 1:29 says:

> *And God said, Behold, I have given you every herb bearing seed, which is upon the face of the earth, and every tree, in which is the fruit of a tree yielding seed; to you it shall be for meat.*

Everything was in perfect health and harmony at that time. Fruits, vegetables, nuts, berries, seeds and flowers were in abundance—this is perhaps the strongest evidence for vegetarianism. Remember also that the air had to have been the purist of pure, as was the water. We have since come close to destroying all the goodness that God has provided us. Was it not His initial intention to have us all live in the Garden of Eden? Is it not His same intention to have us restore on Earth what awaits us in Heaven, when He asks us to pray in Luke 11:2:

When ye pray, say, Our Father which art in heaven, Hallowed be thy name. Thy kingdom come. Thy will be done, as in heaven, so on earth.

As we await the second coming of Christ, it is prophesized in Isaiah 11:6-7:

The wolf also shall dwell with the lamb, and the leopard shall lie down with the kid; and the calf and the young lion and the fatling together; and a little child shall lead them.

And the cow and the bear shall feed; their young ones shall lie down together: and the lion shall eat straw like the ox.

These two verses are a sign to me that we will once again return to vegetarianism. There will be no carnivores or killing of one another as man or beast. We will return to a peaceful coexistence on Earth as it is in heaven. If this was the original plan and if you believe as I do that this is the end plan, whatever happened to us in-between? Shouldn't we be seeing the value of God's wisdom and begin to detach from our indulgent food addictions—such as junk food, soda pop, sugar, fried foods, fast food, as well as meat—and prepare the way for God's Kingdom on Earth?

Whether or not you have a different view of vegetarianism, let's agree that making good dietary changes will improve your health—eating a larger portion of food from a healthfully nurtured garden should be everyone's goal. Eat a strict vegetarian diet if you are in health crisis.

Creating better resources for food...

Today, we could recreate our own "Garden of Eden" at home by growing our own food within a healthy, natural environment—or at least make some attempt to do so, which I will also talk about later.

The best food for you is that which is grown as close to your home as possible because it provides the best immunity and resistance to disease. If you could graze through your gardens, trees and bushes each time you were hungry and eat a varied harvest of seasonally ripe and raw food, you would probably be eating the best diet, provided of course, you constantly built up the fertility of your soil and had clean air and water (more about soil later).

The next best diet would be to grow as much of your own food as possible and then trade/barter with a neighbor or friend to obtain more variety. For most of you reading this book this is certainly challenging, to say the least. However, there are several options to becoming involved in your own food production, and I will go into this in a later chapter where I discuss agriculture. For you avid gardeners who love to grow and have the ability to do so, I would encourage you to do as much as you possibly can to assist others by sharing, bartering, teaching and bringing your excess to market. This is a valuable service for God's Kingdom. More growers-only-farmers-markets are needed in order to obtain local fresh food straight from the source, not from a reseller.

Here is a brief outline of healthy eating that I will cover for you:

- Know exactly where our food comes from and how it was raised—hopefully free from man-made chemicals.
- Eat as much of our food as fresh as possible.
- Use healthy cooking techniques.
- Store food properly and avoid contamination and waste.
- Minimize processed food in our diets prepared outside our own kitchen.
- Read and understand food labels (if you can believe them).
- Learn about acid/alkaline balance in our diet.
- Practice healthy food combining.

Where does our food come from?

Red Hawk, a noted Arkansas poet, who also is a dear friend, tells an American Indian interpretation of the words, "words are not actions" in one of his best poems of the same title. Many ancient cultures used the thoughts expressed by the saying "words are not actions" to measure each other and strangers. In the twenty years that I have been involved in local agriculture, many words have been uttered in support of local farmers but no actions have followed. Most small farmers that I know of have stopped farming, sold out at low land values or downsized because there are not enough local markets for what they grow, and they are not receiving a fair price.

The politics of farming is all too familiar to me since I have much experience in this area. I started out visiting and staying at many small farms in Arkansas because I wanted to learn all that I could about how to grow quality, healthy food. Later, I lived and worked on an Amish farm, as previously mentioned in my introduction, and in 1994 partnered with Dharma Farma organic orchards and gardens in Osage, AR for a period of eight years. I wanted to learn from the master organic orchardist/gardener who was opening his 700-acre farm to selected residents. During this time, Rose and I developed a winter greenhouse research project designed from Eliot Coleman's book, *Four Season Harvest* and marketed mixed fresh salad greens to local health food stores.

My practical knowledge of organic farming and growing concern for the health and dietary habits of people in Arkansas led me to my involvement as a vendor and board member of the Fayetteville Farmers' Market and as president of our state organic grower's association. However, I cannot tell you how frustrating it was to me, as a local farmer, to bring our certified organic, hand picked, tree ripened, heritage apples, pears and cherries to the back dock of the local health food stores and receive only a token order from the produce buyer. The same held true in the winter time with our fabulous salad greens. The large organic produce sections of these stores were filled with non-local produce. Other local growers muttered and complained but were afraid to irk the buyer who would often not buy anything for spite. Natural Health/Food stores, many of which were founded with local community support, sold books proclaiming that eating local food produces local health and then used most of their locally derived income supporting out-of-state food brokers rather than getting to know local farmers.

The inner voice of the Holy Spirit has prodded me most of my life with these words, "If not now, when and if not you, who?" I began to take my case to the board of directors and then to the newspapers. Eventually, I planned a picketing of the store. Rose and I made placard signs on long sticks and tried to get other growers to join us on a busy Saturday, but no others showed up. Now, there is a "new consciousness" about the benefits of local food but money still talks.

Millions of words have been uttered nationally and locally that show support of local farmers, yet produce buyers continue to buy out-of-state or out-of-country produce from large corporate farms by way of big money brokers and truckers even when seasonal, locally grown, lovingly raised food is available. The majority of restaurants with creative chefs still do not create seasonal specialties around local food. Large grocery chains are only interested in convenient delivery at the lowest possible price and some local buyers have been reported to ask for payoffs in order to do business. I suspect that this practice was not unique to Arkansas when I lived there but it prevails today throughout America. If it weren't for the consciousness of a few citizens and communities striving to make a difference, as I and others did then, we might no longer have the option of locally grown food. And more needs to be done. Hopefully, I have incited some of you to demand better choices when it comes to feeding yourself and your families.

The USDA has recently usurped the term "organic" from the small family farmer who nurtured his land with sustainable, chemical-free methods using compost and love. The new government-controlled terminology is "USDA Certified Organic" and is awarded only to growers large enough to afford the large yearly fees. Along with this national standardization and the bureaucracy that runs it arises the inevitable corruption. The best food still comes from small, sustainable, local farms always open to inspection by anyone. In the case of our food supply, bigger is not better—especially now when we are faced with the prospect of having our lifestyles changed by terrorism. Few people realize that stores stock a food supply of only one or two days. This fragile delivery system of our food can be interrupted at any moment. Since so few local family farmers remain, our needs won't be met unless we encourage and revitalize this dying vocation.

What is needed is not only education about the benefits of eating fresh food produced close to home, but also merchants and the public willing to support local growers. A ground swell is beginning to happen nationally. Local growers will hopefully continue to team up with a few pioneering local stores willing to lead the way and provide outlets for fresh local seasonal food. Let us all consider putting words into actions.

What are the benefits of eating "fresh" food?

Let's talk about plant food. We all know that when you bring a bouquet of roses home for your loved one or purchase your favorite, live arrangement for your holiday dining room table, you must keep it watered or in good soil or it will die. When it dies, it loses its vitality—leaves go limp, color fades and it eventually dries up. That beautiful, fresh arrangement will always look best within the first several hours, say 12–24 perhaps, of when you first brought it home.

The same is actually true for our fresh produce when we bring it home from the grocery. The fresher it is when we eat it, the more "live" benefits we derive from it such as vitamins, minerals, proteins and enzymes. Once our produce is harvested, it loses its own life-sustaining forces and so it is gradually dying. The farmer and transporters now need to do everything possible to curtail this dying process or the food will become spoiled before it reaches our tables.

If food is to be shipped over long distances, one option that is most often utilized is to harvest certain crops before they are fully ripened. Have you ever seen or heard the words "vine-ripened" in regards to a desirable fruit or vegetable being sold or applied to the production of a quality wine? Besides questioning the validity of their advertising, one must assume that there should be "added value" to the product they are marketing. Haven't you felt that way? Most agricultural scientists would agree that the most optimum time to pick a fruit or vegetable is when the plant offers the least resistance. In other words it is freed from the vine most easily. This would be when it has reached its full maturity or ripening and would soon fall naturally to the ground. I believe that food picked ripe directly from the garden allows for the development of its full and natural potential and thus is the healthiest to eat. Of course, we do not all have this luxury and so the trucking of large quantities of produce across the country has become big business and another fact of life in our society.

Refrigeration makes long-distance transporting of perishables possible. Foods harvested early are then kept cold to slow the ripening process and later gassed to bring about an unnatural ripening appearance.

What we now need to offset this less-than-desirable food supply is more demand and individual participation in buying from local farmers, developing co-ops among friends and neighbors and an effort to grow something of our own—but more on this later.

Since we have addressed the subject of "fresh" plant food, what about "fresh" meat? Is there such a thing?

In biblical times animals were humanely raised and killed for food. Many large families had one person who was a specialist in the task of killing an animal for food. Special prayers were said before and after the kill. A special razor sharp knife was used to slit the throat producing no pain while the animal was being hugged and stroked. The heart continued to pump the blood out of the animal through the deep cut until the animal quietly and peacefully succumbed. Any meat to be eaten was then washed of blood, trimmed of all fat and salted heavily to draw out any remaining blood then washed of the salt and slowly stewed in liquid. This entire process was called "Kosher" meaning "clean" in Hebrew. Kosher meat today is supposed to be killed and prepped in this manner, if you can trust the butcher. But is this clean meat fresh? I suppose that if it were carefully handled, chilled, and quickly transported from slaughter to your home it might be called fresh? What about aging—a controlled temperature and timed hanging process—or curing by smoking or pickling? These methods may preserve and enhance the texture and/or flavor but is the meat considered any fresher? Is it still living—as a live bouquet or "fresh" vegetable? You be the judge.

There is a huge difference between killing an animal humanely and taking it to the slaughter house today—not only for the animal but also for those who eat its meat. Imagine for a moment how you would feel and react if you were to find yourself walking down a street that dead ends into an alley with no outlet except the same way you came in. Now, imagine that you turn to go out but discover that some unruly looking character is approaching you with a club in hand and there is no time to waste—your body chemistry is going into action. We call this the "flight or fight" syndrome. You are fearful and need to go into emergency mode and act quickly—its do or die!

Adrenaline and other chemicals that the body produces in a state of fear, panic and anxiety are pumped into the blood and delivered to all parts of the body. Similarly, this is the situation of the animal taken to the slaughter house, funneled through long rows or loading chutes and then begining to smell and sense what awaits it at the end of the line. By the time that animal has been killed, its blood is loaded up with these chemicals.

Most of the meat being butchered and packaged for sale at the markets today comes from these same slaughtered animals. Besides having been *overly* fed with grain (loaded with hormones and antibiotics)—to fatten them up before slaughter—they now have added chemicals produced by their own body's defenses. There was no time while the animal was alive for the blood to rebalance itself to a healthier state. These "fight or flight" chemicals come from an emotional state of being. What concerns me is that upon ingestion, we too are taking in more of this emotional state of being which contributes to an increase in feelings of anger and/or anxiety. This is why many serious students with spiritual aspirations refrain entirely from eating meat so as to avoid any emotional impact on their thoughts and actions. Even your pets or animals in the wild, know well enough not to take the life of their prey until after it has played with it or just waited long enough until it had actually relaxed and surrendered to its fate. Then these chemicals have had time to subside and the meat is more desirable.

Albert Einstein was quoted in *What's Wrong with Meat Eating?* by Vistara Parham, as saying, "It is my view that the vegetarian manner of living, by its purely physical effect on the human temperament, would most beneficially influence the lot of mankind."

Let us also take into account this fact: Unlike slow decaying plants, as soon as an animal is killed—due to the coagulation of its proteins and the release of destructive enzymes and substances called ptomaines—rapid decomposition and putrefaction begins to take place. The meat industry tries to mask any discoloration with chemical preservatives that make the meat look red. By the time it makes it to your dining table, who knows what stage of decay it is in? And let's not overlook that animals are frequently infected with diseases which go undetected or are simply ignored. You may be eating part of an animal that had cancer even though the cancerous part was cut away.

So, is there such thing as "fresh" meat, you ask? In my opinion, there really isn't.

What is the harm of eating processed food?

The American Heritage Dictionary defines the word "process" as, "a series of actions, changes, or functions bringing about a result." The end result of processing food is a de-mineralized, de-nutritional, stripped down, altered version of its original form or forms. We may think or are being told that we are getting something new and better because they have had to boost it back up with added nutrients, and they have combined it in such a way as to appeal to our unhealthy cravings—especially with sugar, as well as salt, which often acts as a preservative.

Sadly, we can not fix all the contamination problems affecting our water, food and air supply because it is so complexly money driven that the changes needed might bring everything to a standstill. Big business and the people running it do not want to take a loss in order to make things right. Government standards are routinely not adhered to and no one is being held accountable. So, if you really care about your health and the health of your loved ones, then you will allow the seeds that I and my wife Rose are now planting in you to take root. More personal responsibility and a change in lifestyle making new and better choices for yourself are in order, especially when it comes to processed food. It isn't bad enough that our fresh food may be contaminated due to the water, soil and what is being sprayed on it, but then we resort to processing it and packaging it with additional additives and chemicals and consider this to be nourishment.

One serious source of ill health is nitrates and nitrites. Experts do not agree on how much of these can or should be tolerated. Nitrates produce nitrites which are classified as "free radicals". These destroy many vitamins consumed in your diet thus resulting in vitamin deficiency symptoms. According to Dr. Kelley's Nutritional Program—a key component to my cancer recovery, given to me by Dr. Kelley—"Nitrite reacts with and poisons every enzyme in the body...enzymes are essential for such bodily processes as digestion, metabolism, heart action, and sugar assimilation, to name only a few."

Much can be said about nitrates/nitrites however, my goal here is to heighten your awareness of the danger of over consumption since it is creeping into our lives and our bodies at an ever increasing rate. Although Nitrates are naturally present in our soil, water and food, the Nitrogen Cycle found in nature is being exacerbated by today's agricultural practices that are increasing the environmental concentrations. While authorities attempt to measure how much seeps into our water and our food, the problem lies in the fact that nitrites are increased by heat and other reactions.

"Nitrite is produced from nitrate by microbial action occurring outside or within the body, by the action of heat, by reaction with metals and by reaction with other chemicals", states Dr. Kelley. Thus, when we eat food containing nitrates stored in cans as well as heated, we are producing and ingesting even more nitrites than are already in the food. It is impossible to know how much any individual is being exposed to. The best advice is to avoid nitrates and nitrites whenever possible. Nitrates are being added as a preservative and coloring to most all meat for fresher appeal, but they are especially found in higher concentrations in cured and processed meats such as ham, bacon, sausages, jerky and frankfurters. Not only can nitrates/nitrites be toxic to humans but they also take a toll on our environment and the ecological balance of our rivers and lakes.

At the turn of this century, many mainstream agricultural colleges were receiving grants to help local growers. Their plan was to provide both technical assistance and a physical facility to produce processed food which they called "value added". This plan was to help local farmers receive some value from what they could not sell fresh. Rather than bringing more fresh food to market, they devised a process of artificially "revitalizing" dead food for our consumption. Once again, like modern medicine, we treat the symptoms (loss of farmer income) not the causes (low demand). Fresh non-hybrid food, locally grown without synthetic chemicals using sustainable techniques and consumed without processing is the healthy immunity we all need. The factory farm model of mass production being taught does not fulfill this role. The function of a great university should be to lead in the forefront of education, not follow the corporate dictates of financial benefactors. What kind of graduate is produced by a school of agriculture that has forsaken the small family farmer? What agricultural student would ever want to be a small family farmer when there are no markets that appreciate food raised with love and the nurture of the land?

Fortunately today Farmers' Markets are on the increase along with the desire for fresh, organic produce. An apparent upstart of young married couples or groups of friends is going back to the idea of smaller farm life—working and nurturing the land, simplified lifestyles and the gratification that comes from living off the land as well as putting food on the table for others in their community.

Why is acid/alkaline balance a vital key to health?

Oftentimes, I come across popular books on nutrition that provide some answers for good health, but at the same time overlooks an important component, and by their omission, I feel does just as much harm as good.

To understand human nutrition you must understand acids and alkalies and their relationship to each other. Acids are compounds that have a sour taste and are usually of a corrosive nature. Acids may be classed as either strong or weak and numbers are assigned to the relative strengths. A substance that tends to make an acid solution less acid, or weaker, is an alkali. The symbol "pH" is used to express varying degrees of acidity and alkalinity. Expressions of pH often confuse non-chemists, so a brief explanation here will help.

"pH"

The letters pH stand for "potential hydrogen". The pH scale ranges from 0-14. The midway point, 7.0, is neutral, neither acid nor alkaline. A pH number less than 7.0

indicates acidity. The lower the number is, the stronger the acid. A pH rating above 7.0 indicates the solution's ability to neutralize acids. The higher the number, the stronger it's neutralizing ability. The number 1, therefore, indicates a strong acid and the number 14 indicates a strong alkali. Small differences in pH value represent large differences in acidity or alkalinity, as each whole number represents a ten-fold change in strength. Solutions with a pH of 3.0 are ten times as acid as with a pH of 4.0 and one hundred times as acid as a pH of 5.0. The exact opposite is true on the alkaline scale from 7 to 14.

pH test papers may be helpful in regulating acid/alkali balance. Establish a baseline of testing urine and saliva two hours after the midday meal. ***It should be our goal to achieve 6.4 as the optimum reading indicating our body is in balance.***

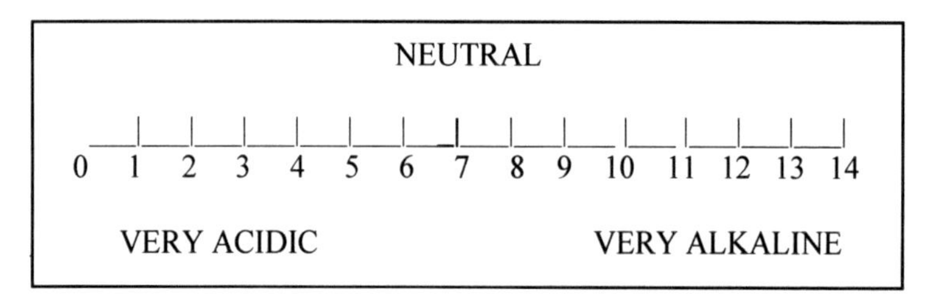

Some foods contain naturally occurring (organic) acids and acid-forming minerals. In general, the acids normally found in food are weak. Two examples of these found in citrus fruits are citric and ascorbic acids, the latter being known as Vitamin C. Other weak, naturally occurring acids are acetic, which gives vinegar its characteristic taste; tartaric, found in grapes and oxalic found in rhubarb, spinach and other vegetable leaves.

Many foods that don't contain acids in their natural state deposit acid-forming minerals in the intestines when digested. These minerals are absorbed by the blood and combine with other elements causing acids to form. If a food is eaten and results in the blood and urine becoming more acidic, the food is termed, “acid-forming”.

The fact that a food contains some naturally occurring acids—such as citric, ascorbic or acetic—does not necessarily make it acid forming. Most fresh fruit and vegetables, in addition to containing small amounts of food-acid, contain high amounts of minerals known to neutralize acids in the blood. These foods are labeled alkaline-forming, not acid-forming. Got it? If not, we'll come back to this shortly.

Acid Body Conditions...

We're all familiar with acid body conditions indicated by sour stomachs, acid indigestion, sour belches and "heartburn" caused by stomach gas. Most of these symptoms are caused by gross errors in diet and are easily correctable. When acids and alkalies are brought together, gas is formed, which disappears when chemical balance has been established. The alkaline reserve is the amount of alkalies available in the blood to neutralize acids at any given time. The higher this reserve, the more resistant is the body to acid conditions forming.

The body is naturally designed to maintain proper balance. Calcium is used as a buffer for over acidity. When there is no reserve to use, the calcium has to be taken from the bone structure itself and especially from teeth in growing children. In adults, it is usually first taken from the spine and pelvic bones—when not replaced, overtime, this leads to osteoporosis. Over-supplementation is not the solution—maintaining a more alkaline diet with weight bearing exercise is.

The chemicals phosphorus, choline and sulfur are all acid forming. Meat, fish, poultry, eggs, cereal, most nuts and legumes are rich in these substances. Alcohol, caffeine and nicotine are acidic.

The chemical elements calcium, potassium, sodium and magnesium are all alkalizing. These are found in fresh, unsulfured fruit and raw vegetables. If there are insufficient alkalies in the diet then blood reserves become exhausted. In order for the body to neutralize an over acidic condition, additional reserves are drawn from bones, bone joints, bone caps, ligaments and/or nerve sheaths. The resulting voids can fill with body fluid (water) resulting in painful inflammation and weakening of the skeletal system and osteoporosis.

The end result of protein digestion and metabolism is largely acidic. For this reason, most nutritionists recommend consuming no more protein than the body needs daily for repair and rebuilding. Excess protein cannot be stored in the body as carbohydrates and fat can. Excess protein must be broken down and the acid wastes eliminated. The resultant drain on alkaline reserves can damage the entire body's metabolism. End products of protein metabolism such as uric acid, sulfuric acid, carbonic acid, etc., require more water to flush these wastes from the blood than does a diet rich in natural carbohydrates and vegetable fat. This is why there is a rapid weight-loss on high protein diets as body tissues give up their fluids to flush out these toxins. When your diet contains too high a proportion of protein in relation to carbohydrates and fat, alkaline minerals are lost every time you urinate and a more acid blood results. Excess protein not broken down and eliminated ends up remaining either in our intestinal tract or in our blood.

Arranging an Alkaline-Ash Diet...

When foods are burned in the body a residue called "ash" is left. The "ash" is the minerals that the food contained. If the minerals: calcium, potassium, sodium and magnesium predominate over phosphorus, chlorine, sulfur and fluorine, then the foods are designated alkaline-forming foods. If the reverse is true, then the foods are designated as acid forming. The excess of one group of minerals over the other found in the ash may be expressed in numbers. The higher the number is, then the higher the acid or alkalizing potential of the food.

The best way to arrange your diet is to consume about 75% of your total daily calories from the alkaline-forming foods and the remaining 25% may then be made up of acid-formers. The fact that a food forms acid does not mean it should be eliminated from your diet or routinely avoided. All protein-containing foods are acid forming, yet protein is essential for life. It is the excesses of these foods that are not required for life, that are to be avoided.

All cereal grains leave acid residues. In addition, processed cereals have lost 50% to 75% of their minerals before you receive them and mandatory enrichment does not add back all of the alkaline minerals lost. This results in increased blood acidity when these grains are frequently eaten. While whole grains are a 100% improvement over processed, they still leave acid reactions.

Milk is often prescribed on an alkalizing diet as being less acid forming than other animal protein foods such as meat, eggs, or cheese. Milk is not a concentrated protein due to its high water content and raw milk and raw milk dairy products leave slightly alkaline reactions. Yogurt and buttermilk made at home from raw milk are also advisable over store bought, pasteurized products—the pasteurization making the foods slightly acid forming.

As you will see, fresh fruits and vegetables form the bulk of an alkalizing diet, but note that fruits which have been candied, jellied, glazed, sugared or sulfured lose their alkaline-forming abilities.

Dried beans are sometimes classed as alkaline-forming, but in general they leave acid reactions due to their high protein contents. Their natural combination of protein and starch also makes them difficult to digest and gas forming. Limit their use and combine them with raw, green salads for the least acid reactions. Hints on cooking beans are found in the next chapter.

The following lists will help you to discern a variety of foods and their pH range for menu planning. The problem is that most people are "hooked" on acidic foods. Whenever Rose and I go out to a restaurant, we can not help noticing that most peoples' plates, even at a Chinese buffet, will look predominately brown in color. Where we would pick out as many varied vegetables as we could, they would load up on the meat and starches. Rose, thinking as an artist, would often tell students to just plan their meals and to arrange their plates with plenty of color and they would be on their way to healthier eating—another very significant reason for this fact is that the different colors in foods are caused by the minerals within.

ACID-FORMING FOODS

Highly Acid-forming:

Refined/ Processed foods
Alcoholic beverages
Margarine
Marmalade

Artificial sweetener	Mayonnaise
Cola-drinks	Nicotine
Caffeine	Refined fats
Candy	Refined sugars
Chocolate	Preservatives, most
Cocoa	Sulfured fruits
Coffee	Syrups
Condiments	Tea, black
Hydrogenated oils	Tobacco
Jams and jellies	Vinegar

Acid-Forming Flesh Foods:

Beef	Ham	Pork
Chicken	Herring	Salmon
Codfish	Lamb	Sardines
Fish, Black	Lobsters	Trout
Haddock	Oysters	Turkey
Halibut Steak	Perch	Veal

Other Animal-Products: Cheese, Eggs, Pasteurized Milk

Other Acid Forming Foods

Nuts: Cashews, Peanuts, Walnuts

Cereal Grains: Barley, Buckwheat, Cornmeal, Millet, Oatmeal, Rice, Rye, Wheat

Vegetables: Jerusalem Artichokes, Brussels Sprouts, Rhubarb, Beans: Kidney; Navy; White

ALKALINE-FORMING FOODS

Alkaline-Forming Fruits

Apples	Guavas	Peaches
Apricots, fresh	Honeydews	Pears

Bananas, yellow
Cantaloupes
Casabas
Cherries
Currants
Grapefruit
Tangerines
Lemons
Loganberries
Mangos
Nectarines
Oranges
Pineapples
Sapodillas
Strawberries
Watermelons

Highly Alkaline Fruits:

Avocados
Bananas, very ripe
Blackberries
Dates
Peaches, dried
Persimmons
Plums
Pomegranates

Very Highly Alkaline Fruits:

Apricots, dried
Figs, dried
Olives, green
Olives, ripe

Alkaline-Forming Vegetables:

Asparagus
Bamboo shoots
Beans, green
Broccoli
Cabbage
Cauliflower
Chicory
Corn, sweet
*Eggplant
Horseradish
Kohlrabi
Leeks
Turnips
Squashes
Lettuce
Mushrooms
Okra
Onions
Parsley
Peas, green
Peas, dried
*Potatoes, white
Potatoes, sweet
*Peppers, green
Pumpkins
Radishes
*Tomatoes
Watercress

*Nightshade family—AVOID on SPECIAL DIETS

Highly Alkaline Vegetables:

Beans, fresh lima
Bean sprouts, soy
Beets
Carrots
Celery
Chives
Cucumbers
Endive
Kale
Onions, dried
Parsnips
Rutabagas

Very Highly Alkaline Vegetables:

Beans, dried	Chard, Swiss	Spinach
Beans, soy	Dandelion greens	Turnip greens
Beet greens	Mustard greens	

Alkaline Dairy: Buttermilk, Milk raw

Alkaline Nuts:	**Very Alkaline Nuts:**
Coconut, fresh	Almonds
Coconut milk, fresh	Chestnuts, fresh
	Chestnuts, dried

Minerals are more important than vitamins...

A loss of minerals is one of the key components to illness. It takes many different minerals to produce the electricity necessary to energize our body. The best way to obtain these minerals is to eat a wide variety of food that has color. Color your plate of food like a rainbow or artists palette. No more than one-quarter should be brown or white food.

The following list will give you some ideas:

Calcium comes from dark leafy green vegetables.
Chlorine comes from unrefined natural salt.
Chromium comes from vegetable oil and whole grain.
Cobalt comes from wheat germ and soy.
Copper comes from raisins and beans.
Fluorine comes from green tea.
Iodine comes from kelp.
Iron comes from beans, wheat germ, raisins and beets.
Magnesium comes from beans, nuts, leafy vegetables, wheat bran and wheat germ.
Manganese comes from bananas and whole grains.

Molybdenum comes from beans and whole grains.
Phosphorus comes from beans and fruit.
Potassium comes from fruit.
Selenium comes from whole grains.
Silicon comes from citrus and whole grains.
Sodium comes from unrefined natural salt.
Sulphur comes from nuts, oats and beans.
Zinc comes from sesame seeds, pumpkin seeds, potatoes and black strap molasses.

The minerals above, plus a myriad of trace minerals too numerous to name but equally important, are also found in whole grains, nuts, seeds vegetables and fruits.

Our best source of food with healthful minerals is from organically grown vegetables from land or sea where no synthetic fertilizers, herbicides, or pesticides have been used. Organic farmers rely on crop rotation, composting of crop residues, cover crops as green manures and biologically safe measures to control insects. Most importantly they encourage soil fertility by enriching its natural minerals with earthworms and natural enzymes.

Many people who are not fond of eating vegetables but concerned about nutrition have either resorted to taking mineral supplements or juicing their vegetables. The latter is the most desirable choice since you are providing the cells of your body with living food. One popular and highly beneficial way to take in your needed minerals is by consuming wheatgrass.

What's so great about wheatgrass?

It's so easy; anyone can grow their own supply of wheatgrass. Its beneficial properties and many diverse uses make this readily and naturally attainable source of nutrition almost a necessity for any personal health and survival kit. Its fiber is indigestible to humans, so it must be juiced for easy consumption—a slow turning juicer is best.

Wheatgrass can provide you with more energy by helping to fill nutritional deficiencies because it contains high quality minerals, vitamins, enzymes and amino acids. It saves you energy. It aids your body's cleansing process by releasing excess fats, mineral deposits and proteins that are trapped in the organs of digestion, elimination and in the blood.

According to Ann Wigmore, who first introduced wheatgrass juice to America over fifty years ago, "Wheatgrass juice is perhaps the most powerful and safest healing aid there is...because it has the ability to strengthen the whole body by bolstering the immune system." She goes on to explain in *The Wheatgrass Book* that Dr. Hans Fischer and a group of associates had won a Nobel Prize for their work on red blood cells. What they discovered was that human blood is practically identical to chlorophyll on the molecular level. Other scientists, working with groups of anemic animals proved that raw, unrefined chlorophyll was able to increase the speed in which new red blood cells were replaced by converting chlorophyll to hemoglobin—strong evidence that wheatgrass juice enriches the blood and supports a healthy immune system that fights off illness.

Living in a world today where the purity of our air, food and water is highly questionable and in some cases, downright toxic, it is vital to know that "chlorophyll can protect us from carcinogens like no other food or medicine can," as Ann Wigmore states. "It acts to strengthen the cells, detoxify the liver and bloodstream, and chemically neutralize the polluting elements themselves," she continues. Further more, studies have shown that chlorophyll-based plants, and especially wheatgrass, can protect us from the damaging effects of all kinds of radiation.

There is no real substitute, however, for growing your own or having someone else do it for you. What you want is a living food—not something in a bottle—and it is recommended that the juice be drunk immediately or it will lose its full potency within fifteen minutes of juicing.

Here is a basic list of what is needed to grow wheatgrass:

1. Find some good topsoil and peat moss or a mixture of topsoil and compost.
2. Purchase some hard plastic trays that can hold 1-inch deep soil.
3. Obtain "hard" or "winter" wheat berries preferably organic.
4. Collect large wide-mouth jars and nylon mesh or open weave cotton cloth to rubber-band over opening for drainage.
5. Have good water and patience.

Here are the basic steps involved in growing wheatgrass:

1. Soak one cup of dry wheat berries in a jar of water for each 10"x14" tray (or more if larger) overnight or for 12 hours.
2. Drain after soaking and rinse well. Retain soaked seeds in the jar at a 45°angle, screened-lid down for 12 hours until berries sprout
3. Spread a smooth, even layer of soil 1-inch thick in a tray allowing for small trenches to catch excess water.

4. Spread the sprouted wheat evenly over the soil with your hands with seeds touching but not overlapping.
5. Sprinkle with water to moisten but do not drench.
6. Cover with a second tray to block out light and set aside for 2–3 days.
7. Uncover and re-water and place in indirect light—growth should be about 1-inch, sturdy, white or yellowish in color.
8. Continue to keep moist with regular watering. In 6–12 days it will be ready to harvest at 7–10 inches tall. Cut close to the soil for concentrated nutrients.

Much more can be said here for the many benefits and uses of wheatgrass in our health arsenal today but I will encourage you to seek out one of the books listed in my bibliography or search online for detailed instructions for growing your own and juicing it on a regular basis. However, like anything else, I am not proposing that wheatgrass be a substitute for a proper detoxification cleansing program or an improved nutritional diet. It is not another "quick fix" all by itself, but when used in concert with a healthy lifestyle, it will boost your results and create an extra layer of protection. Many people can attest to the fact that it has helped them to be healed of cancer.

What a Mother Eats Determines the Health of Her Child and of her family

Just as it says in the Book of Matthew verse 7:17:

Even so every good tree bringeth forth good fruit; but a corrupt tree bringeth forth evil fruit.

We need to look at two important factors here. First is that the mother or primary food provider of the family plays a critical role in determining the health of the family.

Second is that a newborn infant receives his/her best start in life from its mother.

I cannot emphasize enough that any female considering pregnancy should cleanse her body of impurities and begin a diet that will produce the healthiest baby possible. If the developing baby in the womb of the mother is not receiving what he/she needs to feed its growth from the mother's diet alone then the baby will start to draw upon the healthy reserves of the mother, causing her health to decline. If the mother is in poor health at the time of conception and eats a nutritionally deprived diet, both the baby and the mother will suffer. If you are serious about having the healthiest child possible then both the father and the mother need to cleanse their bodies and begin a healthful diet that will produce a healthy baby.

Family members should all be on the same page when it comes to diet. However, if the family is routinely eating a diet that is perceived as unhealthy by one member trying to restore their health, then that person either has to convince the others to change or set themselves apart. A Christian family that recognizes God as the supreme authority also should live by God's plan for the family. The father is designated as the head of the family and should be the final authority on all decisions after listening to everyone's viewpoint. Authority brings a great responsibility to be a role model. In many households, the wife has the sole responsibility for food management and diet. This does not necessarily have to be so as the best chefs are men and it is not feminine to enjoy cooking. I say this, of course, in defense of myself as I am the food management person in our house not only because of my professional restaurant experience but also because I love serving others by properly feeding them.

In most families, food preparation follows a familiar routine that goes back at least one or two generations. We become addicted to certain foods from the womb on to death in most cases. Men usually are addicted to their mama's cooking and girls cook just like mama. When a marriage occurs there may be a clash of tastes unless both parties were raised in the same culture. The children eat what is served. In this typical household everyone will resist a change of diet.

When illness occurs within the family the seeds of that or similar illnesses are in the whole family—as long as they eat the same diet and live the same lifestyle. If illness forces one family member to cause a change for the better, then it may be considered a message and a blessing to the rest of the family because they need to change too.

So, I encourage the one who manages the food in the home to take these words to heart—make a difference for yourselves and for your family by setting a good example and leading others to wellness.

What is meant by "food combining"?

The principle behind food combining is that different classes of food require different enzyme secretions and digestive pH for their digestion. They also have different rates of digestion. In other words, our digestive system is designed to work a particular way so when we eat a variety of foods indiscriminately our digestive system performs inefficiently and this leads to putrefaction, fermentation, toxic acids and heartburn. Researchers and nutritionists have come to recognize that indigestion for many people is the direct result of eating certain foods too closely together, resulting in acid reflux or gas. Antacids are one of the biggest profit making over-the-counter remedies sold in

America and elsewhere today. If you experience these symptoms on a regular basis consider making the following adjustments:

1. Eat fresh fruit alone and allow at least ½ hour for it to leave your stomach before introducing another food type.
2. Do not combine fresh and dried fruit.
3. Do not combine sweet and sour fruit.
4. Eat melons alone.
5. Protein (especially of animal origin) and starch like potato, rice, pasta, and bread are harder to digest when combined together unless the largest portion of the meal is vegetables.
6. Chew all food to mush before swallowing and do not mix with any liquid, drink ½ hour before or after meals.

Another important point of interest is that scientific evidence has proven that when eating live or raw food, the common "food combining" theory of enzyme secretions canceling each other out during the digestive process is much less an issue: the reason being that raw food comes complete with its own specific live enzymes for digestion that are mostly destroyed in cooking. Not only do you get more nutritional benefits from raw food but they also aid our digestion and provide good fiber.

Then there are the predigested foods that occur by soaking or sprouting seeds, nuts or grains which then become much easier to digest and to assimilate. Naturally, if ones diet is primarily raw and predigested food there is less need for concern of proper food combining and preventing indigestion. However, any amount of over-eating—even if all you eat is one type of food—will result in digestive problems. Become your own food detective and pay attention to the signs: gas, constipation or diarrhea, bloating, nausea, or exhaustion after eating. These signs tell us that we need to avoid certain combinations and the quantities consumed in any one meal.

To Eat or Not To Eat, this is the question?

This book would not be complete if I did not address the issue of "clean" versus "unclean" meats as it pertains to God's dietary laws. As I have said before, God has been my inspiration for writing this *Health and Survival Guide*. Why did I subtitle it this way?

First and foremost, it was because I was concerned about health—your health. Having learned from experience how to be healed naturally of cancer, I wanted to empower others to be able to do the same and much, much more since what I have discovered applies not only to cancer but to any illness affecting the body. The body's ability to heal itself is set in motion by a person making these same choices and using these simple self-administered techniques I have described. The choices are yours to make because God gave us all the freedom of choice. You can achieve good health for yourself and set an example for your friends and loved ones by choosing a healthier lifestyle for yourself as I have done.

Along the way, I have encountered obstacles that I have had to overcome and so will you. I needed to unlearn much of what I was taught in medical school in regard to treating just the symptoms of a health problem with medications and/or surgery. I had to overcome my aversion to giving myself enemas, and I had to drastically (at least while my body was in crisis) change my diet. At the time, giving up certain foods definitely did seem drastic because I had become addicted to what I was used to eating. My cravings and whatever was conveniently available to me in restaurants and at the supermarkets took precedence over any sound logic that had either been handed down to me by my mother, acquired from well-wishing friends, picked up by chance from some form of mass media, or lo and behold, found in the truth of the Bible. More often than not, we all refuse to pay attention to advice that is contrary to our own behavior. However, my life really depended on my being willing to change.

Your health may also be in crisis or it may not be but sooner or later it probably will, unless you take the necessary steps to prevent it from happening. Most people I now encounter do not come to me for advice unless they feel their back is up against the wall. Unfortunately, some people wait until their health challenges become a huge uphill battle instead of taking on easier goals that will steadily improve their quality of life. Naturally, we are not meant to live in our physical body forever but I strongly believe that we need to take care of our precious "Temple of God" in order to fulfill the life and purpose that God intended for each of us and to receive and enjoy His promised rewards.

The question of "survival"…

It goes without saying, that most people of this world today are concerned about their very survival. There is so much going on at present that is a threat to our lives—such as the effects of global warming and its influences on natural disasters and world food production; loss of income and rising health costs; possible terrorist attacks, and the increase and rapid spread of viruses and bacteria that could lead to a worldwide pandemic. But, if you have faith in God as I do, then you might not be as worried as some others are. Certainly, devout Christians firmly believe that their salvation is assured and their fate predetermined according to God's plan so why make an effort to improve and maintain your health? They say to me, "Why bother to change anything when we should instead just accept our lot in life?" I have come across this attitude among many of my sisters and brothers in Christ. Since God gave us free choice to love and obey Him or not, then the degree to which we decide to follow His example is up to each one of us. I sincerely believe God never intended for His children to suffer and to be inflicted with illness. According to 3 John: 2:

> *Beloved, I wish above all things that thou mayest prosper and be in health, even as thy soul prospereth.*

The truth is we bring illness on ourselves. The choices we make—whether or not we hold ourselves to God's Law —all have consequences. If you are an orthodox Jew, then you take God's dietary laws spoken of in Deuteronomy and Leviticus very seriously. Otherwise, you may consider yourself to be a Jew but pretty much eat as you please. If you call yourself a Christian, than you are probably thinking right now that by the grace of God you are no longer held accountable to God for these Old Testament laws. Well, I do not claim to be a theologian or a minister of the Gospel but I have been examining this controversial question of what to eat or not to eat for some time now. My studies have revealed to me that too many believers have taken God's words out of context and turned them into a misconception because it is more agreeable and convenient to think that way. Let me reiterate what I spoke of in the preface of this guide book: one's salvation in the Kingdom of God may be assured but one's health in their body while on earth is not and must be earned. We have been made custodians of the dwelling place of His Spirit. Is this not a sacred trust? The Lord also declares in Hosea 4:6:

My people are destroyed for lack of knowledge; because thou hast rejected thee, I will also reject thee, that thou shalt be no priest to me: seeing thou hast forgotten the law of thy God, I will also forget thy children.

Are we to ignore His Word and pay a price in the Heavenly Kingdom as well? These questions are too often avoided today when it comes to our diets.

We need to ponder the fact that God doesn't lie and that all of His wisdom, whether it is found in the Old Testament or New Testament is in our best interest so that we may maintain a healthy body, mind and spirit and live fruitful lives in His eyes. My purpose, here, is not to convince you of what I think you ought to do but rather to enable you to more closely understand what God is telling us. When I was working at the Nutritional Clinic in Leslie, Arkansas, I came in contact with a few particular books that have greatly influenced me. One of these is called *God's Key to Health and Happiness*, written by Elmer A Josephson, an ordained Baptist Minister whose own serious illnesses were cured by following the Bible teachings he later felt compelled to share with others in his book. What captivated me was the following quote from the Bible and his response to it:

Apostle Paul says in I Timothy verse 4:

For every creature of God is good, and nothing to be refused, if it be received with thanksgiving.

More often than not, this verse is interpreted to mean that every creature of God is good and not considered “unclean” to eat just as long as you are thankful for it—the emphasis being on “every creature”. And, since all creatures are created by God, Elmer Josephson states, “This would include every poisonous reptile, venomous serpents, and deadly vipers, even to the wriggling mass of loathsome maggots and worms that feed on dead rotten carcasses. Not only so, but it would be approving cannibalism, the eating of humans. We, of course, know that this is not the case.”

He goes on to illustrate that God is not distinguishing between those He created and those He did not create. If you believe in Creation, then that idea is nonsensical. He then substitutes the phrase, “Every man of God is worthy to be received into your home”. If we apply the same reasoning, then we see that “every man” would be welcomed by you into your home. Speaking for myself, I certainly would not permit just any man or woman into my home. We are not all righteous in our actions. So, instead, what we really need to discern here and focus on is the phrase “of God”. We need to keep in mind that in Bible times, “God’s people distinguished between the clean and unclean, the holy and unholy, that which was ‘of God’ and that which was not. They never held the unclean and unholy to be ‘of God’.” This is a key point that Elmer Josephson is making here. If we take a look at Leviticus 2: 44 which says:

> *For I am the Lord your God: ye shall therefore sanctify yourselves, and ye shall be holy; for I am holy: neither shall ye defile yourselves with any manner of creeping thing that creepeth upon the earth.*

The word "sanctify" does not mean to pray over. What it does mean is "to set apart". Sound familiar? The Word of God clearly identifies in Leviticus 2 and Deuteronomy 14 (the chapters containing God's dietary laws) which meats are sanctified as clean and which are not. These sanctified meats are therefore spoken of as "of God". I am confident that in God's ultimate wisdom that He had very good reason for this and we would greatly benefit if it were still applied today. The choice is ours to make. Unfortunately our intelligence and faith in God's wisdom is hampered by a manipulating world mentality. If you were to break another of God's Commandments—let's say, you were to steal from your neighbor—no amount of prayer will justify an immoral action and make right what is wrong. So, while a prayer of thankfulness is a good idea, it will not make your dietary choices more healthful in the eyes of God and you must decide for yourselves how obedient are you willing to be.

Elmer Josephson goes on in his book to refute many other interpretations of God's Word that have been widely accepted for their literal meaning and not looked at in their correct context. I highly recommend people to read it. For my purposes, I will just leave you to chew on this one commentary for a while.

Nobody knows for sure what our survival rate will be in the "end times" —considered by many Christians, today, to have already begun. How long will it last? What conditions will each of us have to endure? The answers are yet to unfold. Will we perish, become stricken with disease, be taken up in the "rapture" by God, or left behind to serve Him in some special capacity? Are we preparing ourselves, ever watchful and ready for the return of Christ? Of course, our God is a loving and merciful God and continues to offer us opportunities for redemption. This leads me to ask: Are we living just to eat, or are we eating so that we may honor God? How far are we willing to go to set ourselves apart"?

Many of you may be considering that this is the time to incorporate some changes into your life. Let me just say that, for most of you, this is not an overnight process unless you are currently dealing with an acute illness. Most changes occur over time and as you notice the benefits you will be encouraged to make other changes. Personally, I have gone from a carnivorous and out-of-balance diet to a strict vegetarian diet and then to what I call a "flexitarian" diet—this is when, for years, I would only indulge in meats and certain other foods when I had to eat out at a friend's house or at a restaurant. This approach enabled me to "fit in" and not be stressed on these occasions—an especially good time to exercise the act of prayer over my food. However, having recently been exposed to Dr. Colin Campbell's book, *The China Study*, I am convinced that the best diet is a plant-based diet with no exceptions. My wife and I, once again, are turning over a new leaf.

Before moving on from this subject, I would like to leave you with some thoughts as to why pork and shell fish, ravenously enjoyed in our culture today, are considered "unclean" from a practical stand point. First of all, they are scavengers in that they will eat anything and everything and thus act as waste disposals. They eat the slop and the dead things settling in the ocean, respectively.

Pigs are omnivores, eating both plant and animal food. Their digestive tract is most like ours which takes a much longer period to process food for utilization as opposed to a carnivore that only eats meat and food passes through their system more quickly. This longer process of digestion only adds to the contamination of the ingested food, since there is more time for putrefaction to take place in the intestinal tract. Any undigested food residue is a breeding ground for bacteria that causes yeast, viruses and parasites to multiply. Now, you may be saying, "But what if these pigs are farm raised and well fed?" Well, a pig's flesh is most like ours too in that fat is distributed throughout its' meat and can not be cleanly cut away when prepared or served. Toxins which are mostly stored in fat are then saturated within the meat and can not be avoided when devoured. One might go so far as to say that eating a pig's flesh is most akin to cannibalism because of the similarities in the way we process food and store the end results.

I believe that we were intended to be herbivores although we have mostly become omnivores and our own inability to digest meat properly has led to all kinds of health problems that begin with the need for that quick over-the-counter remedy and then lead to more serious problems down the road.

That fresh-caught lobster, just brought in from the ocean, has been living on dead debris all of its life as do all shell fish. God did not intend for us to survive on dead tissue and waste from other sea creatures. There is an old saying, "You are what you eat". We used to laugh at this when we were kids but it isn't very far from the truth. The building blocks these creatures rely on for their bodily functions are not the same building blocks our physical body needs to survive on. On the contrary, we need live enzymes available in fruits and vegetables for good digestion and naturally supplied nutrients in living food for good health.

So, what about farm-raised lobster, shrimp and crab, you say? These creatures are being fed a man-made feed, kind of like your dry dog food, that contains both artificial coloring, and pharmaceutical drugs…enough said.

If you really want to read the most convincing and scientific evidence on the subject of animal protein and your health I urge you to obtain a copy of *The China Study* by T. Colin Campbell.

I end this section with this thought from Corinthians 6:20:

> *For ye are bought with a price: therefore glorify God in your body, and in your spirit, which is God's.*

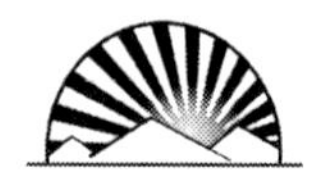

Chapter Five: **Healthy Food Preparation… Tips from a Chef**

Here's where I get to put on my chef's hat and apron…as a creature of habit, my wife can tell you, I am never preparing food without one.

I have had the privilege to work with a few of the best chefs. In 1980 I was working as an assistant chef under Executive Chef, Brother Ron Picarski. Brother Ron, a Francescan monk, was hired by the award winning Unicorn Village Restaurant in N. Miami Beach, Fl. after being awarded the Gold Medal in the Cooking Olympics held in Belgium. It was a real privilege to have worked with him. He used vegan creations to outdo world class chefs. Brother Ron and other great chefs were a real inspiration to me. My love of cooking and forty-year pursuit of nutritional health inspires me now to emphasize to others the importance of certain techniques of food preparation, food storage and basically what a well-stocked kitchen and pantry ought to have on hand.

To condense so vast a subject into some form that can easily be digested mentally and physically is a daunting task.

In terms of living enzymes, the healthiest food is acquired by feasting from your own organic garden. Cooking most vegetables as little as possible is the goal to preserving living enzymes. I cannot emphasize strongly enough that, in my opinion, the best overall lifestyle is to return to the family farm, a small rural community way of life. Living close to the land and practicing sustainability brings a consciousness not found in urban settings. Perhaps, the only exception that I know of is in Cuba, where in 2002, there were 35,000+ organic vegetable gardens in and around Havana.

We are going to begin with lists of items to acquire over time, as you are able. Please note that a microwave should ***not*** even be in your home as we have discussed in chapter two. Another item that I strongly discourage the use of is aluminum foil when used for cooking, e.g. baking potatoes. Foods prepared with aluminum foil absorb aluminum—studies have shown that an excess of non-plant based aluminum (also found in most antiperspirants) is detrimental to our health and contributes to Alzheimer's disease. Aluminum naturally occurring in plants however is harmless.

Kitchen Utensils etc., *listed as close to the order of importance as we can come:*

1. "Big Berkey" counter top, gravity water purifier is your best investment for water you can trust.
2. Professional chef knives, and sharpening steel or stone. When I was a lowly prep cook working with veteran chefs, I learned by observation. For many years the best knives were considered German and that was what I bought. When Rose married me she had a set of professional knives from France which, at first, I disdained, but now admit they are as good as or better than my German knives. Quality working tools are a sound investment.
3. Hardwood cutting board or two—as large as your counter space will allow.
4. Norwalk or Green Star juice extractor

5. Wooden, ceramic and stainless steel bowls, large, medium and small
6. Professional rubber spatula and heat resistant silicon spatula
7. Cast iron skillets with lids, large and small
8. Cast iron griddles, round and rectangular covering two burners
9. Stainless steel 18/8 or better saucepans with vapor seal lids, very large, large, medium, and small
10. Stainless or carbon steel skillets with lids, large, medium, small
11. Large covered wok, carbon or stainless steel
12. Large stainless steel strainer or colander and small stainless steel strainer
13. Measuring cups and spoons
14. Wooden spatulas, spoons, fork, 4-inch stainless-steel spatula
15. Hand-crank can opener
16. Stainless steel swivel peeler
17. Wire cheese cutter (optional.)
18. Small toaster oven (optional.)
19. Blender/grinder
20. Stainless steel hand grater
21. Stainless steel wire whip (whisk) medium and small
22. Attractive plates, bowls and serving pieces
23. Large white professional bib aprons and utility towels

Stocking the Larder…

These basic provisions should always be on hand and then supplemented with a variety of fresh foods whenever possible. Again we try to list these in the order of their importance and recommend organic if possible.

1. Extra Virgin cold pressed olive and/or coconut oil in cans (light destroys nutrients)
2. Salad greens and cooking greens
3. Fresh garlic and ginger
4. Carrots, celery, parsley, lemons/limes
5. Peppers, hot and sweet
6. Potatoes , sweet potatoes and green cabbage
7. Onions and any in-season vegetables
8. Tomatoes, tomato paste (Del Monte with nothing added)
9. Celtic sea salt is an *extremely* beneficial supplement to your diet as it contains multiple minerals and trace minerals and is in my opinion the best salt in the world right now. Sources are Selina or Salt Works
10. Spike salt-free seasoning
11. Cayenne pepper
12. Oregano, basil, paprika, chili powder, coriander, cinnamon, allspice and cancer-fighting spices such as cumin, ginger and turmeric. Use fresh, not bottled, whenever possible.
13. Soft, raw milk cheese and cow butter (optional)
14. Fresh, free range, fertile eggs (optional)
15. Short- and long-grain brown rice, rolled oats, whole grain pastas
16. Raw almonds, pecans, walnuts, sunflower seeds, pumpkin seeds
17. Aged wheat-free tamari or Braggs Liquid Aminos
18. Serenity Farm or sprouted bread (whole grain, non baker's yeast only)
19. Dried lentils, peas and other beans
20. Almond butter (peanuts are notorious for mold and fungus)
21. Green tea
22. Raisins
23. Dried and canned soups
24. Frozen vegetables

25. Sardines packed in unsalted water (optional)
26. Tempeh or Tofu (optional)
27. Fresh in-season and frozen fruits, non-sweetened jams
28. Whole-wheat flour and berries for milling and sprouting
29. Corn meal or corn for milling
30. Honey and maple syrup

Patterns of Eating…

Most people tend to eat on the run, especially in the mornings. Too often, one may skip breakfast entirely or grab something that may give quick energy but is not sustaining. By mid-morning or sooner, one may feel in a slump, have difficulty concentrating, and are looking for another quick fix to keep going till lunch. I believe that ***Breakfas***t is your most important meal of the day. It sets the tone and gives you energy to start your day and to keep your engine going until your next meal. The more active you are the more calories you burn. So, why drain yourself when you need to fuel your body the most? Even the cells of your brain require nourishment. To be your best on the job or do your best in school, you must provide your physical body with the resources it needs to succeed. The bigger the meal, the later in the day or evening, the more energy is required for digestion and fewer calories are burned because you are starting to slow your activity down. When we compensate in the evening for what we deprived ourselves of during the day, it takes a toll on our system and interferes with what should be a restful sleep upon retiring. The word itself is "break-fast". In other words, you are breaking a fast from your last meal. The fast needs to be for twelve hours every day from your last meal (supper) until you break fast. This nightly fast will be a time of healing for your body.

In my opinion, you should ***eat breakfast like a king***. That is to say large and full of nourishment to carry you through to lunch five hours later. My current breakfast, when we are home, is a three-day rotation. The first morning is cooked, organic rolled oats with raisins, a dash of Celtic salt and cinnamon, a little olive oil and three cups water to one cup oats. This is brought to a boil over medium heat, stirring occasionally, then, let stand covered with heat off for five minutes before serving. If you like it a bit thicker, than wait a little longer. I measure ½ cup oats per person or serving and cook this porridge with more liquid to avoid the need for some kind of "milk". With this substantial bowl of porridge, we usually have two slices of whole grain bread grilled with olive oil on a cast iron griddle then sprinkled with cinnamon.

The second breakfast is shredded white potato and carrot mixed with diced onion, tomato and pepper (or use any leftover veggies) plus ¼ cup corn meal grilled with olive oil on a cast iron griddle seasoned with paprika, cayenne and Celtic salt accompanied with grilled whole grain bread.

The third breakfast is whole grain pancakes with fruit compote. Mix two cup whole grain flour with ¼ cup corn meal and ¼ cup rolled oats. Add ½ teaspoon Celtic salt and ½ teaspoon baking soda. Add two tablespoons olive or coconut oil and stir in enough water to make a thin batter. Pour onto lightly oiled, hot griddle making about twenty-four, three-inch diameter small cakes. Turn once when slightly crisp around the edges and bubbly on top. In a small saucepan combine diced fresh fruit of choice, honey, cinnamon and enough water to bring mixture to boil and simmer five minutes before serving over pancakes. Chopped nuts may be added before serving for more nutrition. Often times we top these cakes with warmed, leftover vegetables instead of fruit. Also, we use these pancakes as yeast-free bread for other meals or snacks. They are great re-grilled with a little spicy tomato sauce with garlic and basil.

Next, you should ***eat lunch like a prince***. It is your second most important meal and should be large and substantial enough to hold you five hours until a light supper. Here are some ideas for a three day lunch rotation. Day one will be steamed brown rice, stir-fried vegetables and beans. Also prepare grated fresh beets with diced cucumber, onion, a dash of Celtic salt, lime juice and a little olive oil or a slaw of cabbage, grated carrot, diced onion/pepper etc. Add to this meal fresh sliced avocado with Celtic salt and some lime. Make enough of everything and refrigerate extra for day two and three.

The second lunch is veggie-burgers or loaf with a sauce. Combine the previous rice, beans and vegetables in a large bowl. Then add some rolled oats, corn meal, a little olive oil and paprika. If I did not cook beans previously, then I will add sunflower seeds or chopped nuts instead. Mix thoroughly with a large spoon. Pre-heat and lightly oil a cast iron griddle then drop two large spoonfuls of mixture on griddle for each burger and flatten with a spatula. Use three spoonfuls for a thicker loaf. Reduce heat to low and brown on one side before turning. Make a sauce of Del Monte tomato paste (there is nothing added on their label), Celtic salt, oil, dry mustard, chili powder, cumin and water. Heat and simmer five minutes before spooning over burger/loaf. Complete lunch with more beet salad and avocado as yesterday. Save leftover burgers and sauce for tomorrow.

On day three take yesterday's leftover burgers and break them up in a large skillet. Add the leftover sauce and water. This then becomes a "meat sauce" for your pasta. Cook pasta of choice and then add contents of skillet to sauce and simmer slightly before serving with more beet salad and sliced fresh avocado or a fresh garden salad of choice.

Finally, you should ***eat supper like a pauper***. It should be very light so that when you go to bed, your body is healing not digesting. Our supper consists of a bowl of fresh cut fruit about 4–5 PM, then some green tea with grilled herb bread one hour later. We have our breakfast at 7 AM, so we do not eat after 7 PM.

People tell me that they are not especially hungry in the morning, so they skip or put off breakfast. This is because they are consuming too much food before they go to bed. When your body doesn't need or use the calories taken in it begins to store fat. I think that one of the biggest reasons for people becoming overweight is this daily habit of eating their biggest meal later in the day or worse yet, late in the evening. Believe me, when I say that if you eat your meals as I have recommended you will wake up with a good appetite for breakfast and a fresh start for the day, fueling your body as needed and not overloading it at night. Bedtime should be a time for rest and healing and not for heavy, energy consuming digestion. This change alone could add years to your life.

The importance of chewing...

How many times have you heard your mother or someone else say, "Chew your food before swallowing"? I know that I did many times while growing up. Why is it that we too often forget this good advice and down our food instead with gulps of liquid—soda pop, milk, and juice or even with water?

The "Mayr" method described in Appendix G (Concluding the Seven-Day Cleanse) is very helpful in retraining yourself to eat and chew more consciously. Proper digestion begins in the mouth. Chewing produces saliva that releases digestive juices to begin the process. This action also stimulates other digestive enzymes to be released in the stomach in preparation for the food on its way down to be further digested. The body requires energy to produce these enzymes. So, the more we chew before swallowing, the less energy is needed to further digest what we eat. You are aiding the digestive process. Furthermore, by not diluting your digestive juices with liquid, they are better able to do their job and fewer enzymes are required. As we get older, we lose our ability to more effectively produce these enzymes so what, how and even when we eat really comes into play. We need to learn good eating habits early in life and practice them continually. This way, we will receive the nutrition needed to produce energy for life from our food and avoid indigestion and heartburn, weight gain and other complications. I hope that you will think of me the next time you eat and remember me telling you to "chew your food, the stomach has no teeth". You will begin to enjoy what you eat much more as well.

Healthful Meals…

Once again, the best rule to follow is to eat as fresh as possible, grown as close to your home as possible, organically grown and cooked as little as possible. When planning your menu remember your pH balance. The following hints are for some basic techniques.

Twelve Hints for Healthful Eating

1. A large, ***fresh green salad*** should be the basis of at least one meal daily with various other things added, cooked or raw. I encourage you to make a simple dressing of your own and to avoid some unhealthful and unnecessary additions to bottled dressings. Rose prefers to squeeze some fresh lime juice, a pinch of Celtic salt and some extra virgin olive oil into our salad mixes. Be creative and try adding some finely chopped garlic or ginger. Here in Belize, we like the added zest of some "Marie's Green Habanera Sauce" added to a garden vegetable slaw.

2. ***Cooked vegetables*** can be prepared by cutting into bite-sized pieces. Prepare before beginning to cook. The size of the cut piece should be thicker for softer veggies and thinner for harder veggies to make them cook evenly or veggies can be added to the pan beginning with the hardest first. Dice fresh garlic and onion. The sauté method is as follows: Warm skillet, add olive oil—don't let oil smoke—then garlic, onion and small amount of water. Let cook on medium heat for a couple of minutes and then add other veggies in order of their density, cooking the hardest first. Add seasonings and more liquid if desired, such as a little tomato sauce or broth, cover and simmer until tender but not mushy. Lentils or precooked beans can be added for extra protein.

The ***wok*** method uses the principle of "hot wok, cold oil": Heat wok over high heat until hot. Add about ½ cup olive oil and immediately add the veggies and about another ¼ cup of water or broth to prevent the oil from smoking. Stir quickly to coat all veggies and to seal in juices, season, and place a tight lid on wok, keeping high heat to steam and tenderize for just a few minutes so that veggies are slightly crisp.

3. ***Brown rice*** can be added to your salad or used in different ways. Add two cups purified water for each cup of rice in a saucepan with vapor seal lid. Bring to boil over medium heat, then, reduce to simmer for 45–50 minutes or until bottom of rice is dry. Do not remove lid until final test for dryness with a fork. Remove from heat and allow it to stand covered for five minutes. Turn upside down into wooden bowl, fluff with fork and add a small amount of butter or olive oil to prevent grains sticking and perhaps a dash or two of Braggs Liquid Aminos. Rice can be eaten steamed or cooked in the skillet with olive oil and veggies etc. Small pieces of raw vegetables can be added to the rice before cooking and, when cooked together, create a different taste. This is called a rice pilaf.

4. ***Pasta*** can be added to your salad or used in different dishes with cooked veggies as the sauce. Experiment with different varieties of organic pastas but harder wheat such as Durum is preferred. Add dried pasta to rapidly boiling water in a large enough saucepan. Reduce heat to medium while stirring frequently with a wooden fork to prevent sticking, then, simmer until "al dente"—firm not mushy. Drain in a stainless strainer, return to the pot off the heat and add a small amount of olive oil, toss and eat.

5. ***Nuts*** are a good source of protein and other nutrients. They can be eaten raw, soaked over night

or slightly roasted to kill mold. Almonds are the most healthful. Raw nuts can be spread in a shallow pan and placed in a small toaster oven at 300° until you can smell them, pay attention. Or you can toast nuts/seeds in a cast iron skillet on top of the stove. Then empty into wooden bowl, sprinkle with a small amount of tamari or Braggs Liquid Aminos, and toss until the sizzle stops. Be sure to chew nuts slowly and thoroughly. Nuts can also be blended with water to create a nut milk or heavy cream for sauces or casseroles. Nuts can also be soaked overnight, seasoned and placed in a dehydrator.

Avoid peanuts because they are notorious carriers of mold colonies and fungus. In *The China Study*, T. Colin Campbell, emphasizes that there has been considerable evidence to show that peanuts are often contaminated with a fungus-produced toxin called "aflatoxin"—the most potent chemical carcinogen ever discovered. We need to re-evaluate our fixation with eating and feeding our kids peanut butter and jelly sandwiches (also sugar loaded) while on the go and in our school cafeterias.

6. ***High quality eggs*** are an excellent source of protein and other nutrients but not for people with cancer or illness. By high quality, I mean from free ranging chickens that are allowed to intermingle with a rooster so that the eggs are fertile. Eggs are most healthful soft boiled, with the white somewhat firm and the yellow soft. Whatever your choice, cook them easy. They can be added raw to vegetable rice or pasta casseroles before cooking.

7. Slightly aged, ***raw milk cheese*** such as Colby and raw milk butter are excellent sources of protein, calcium and other nutrients used in moderation. But not for people with cancer or illness.

8. A slice of ***whole grain bread*** grilled with olive oil on a cast iron griddle until slightly brown on both sides can be eaten alone or topped with a thin slice of cheese, tomato, cooked veggies, etc. This bread is also great toasted then spread with crunchy almond butter or simply seasoned with cayenne, Celtic salt and basil. Sometimes we use any leftover morning pancake as a bread re-grilled in the evening with herbs and/or tomato sauce

9. Cooked ***whole rolled oats*** is an excellent source of fiber and nutrition. Add 1½ cup purified water for every ½ cup serving of rolled oats in a covered saucepan. Add a dash of Celtic sea salt, and small amount of butter or olive oil and or raisins if desired. Cook over medium heat until boil, stirring frequently. Then, cover and reduce to simmer for 3 minutes. Turn off heat and let stand for five minutes. Most whole grains, such as quinoa, can be cooked as a breakfast cereal. Grains can be combined raw in several combinations and eaten soaked in liquid like a raw granola or muesli.

10. ***Potatoes*** or ***any vegetable*** can be washed, dried, brushed or rubbed with olive oil then baked at 425° in toaster oven for one hour, turning half way. Or, cut into small pieces and add to stir-fry or grate and brown slightly in a cast iron skillet with olive oil and onions. Or, steam them—cut into small pieces, place in a saucepan with a small amount of water, cover

and bring to boil over medium heat, then simmer holding vapor until tender, then mash with olive oil and or butter and Celtic salt or eat as is.

11. ***Sprouting seeds and grains*** produces live fresh food. However, mold can quickly accumulate on fresh sprouts producing unwanted health problems. Careful techniques must be employed (which we will not attempt to cover here) to prevent mold on all kinds of food.

12. ***A colorful variety of fresh fruits*** supplement your diet with needed vitamins and minerals. Include some daily but even a natural sugar should be eaten in moderation or avoided all together when on a strict cleansing diet. Fruits digest quickly and easily when taken on an empty stomach at least thirty minutes before a meal or at least one hour after a meal or longer if meat is included. When eaten in combination with other foods, it won't break down properly and will likely ferment and cause indigestion. Papaya and pineapple are an exception since they provide extra digestive enzymes.

13. ***Rotation of fresh food*** is critical for not only maintaining health but also for preventing waste. The fresher the food the more alive and nutritionally beneficial it is. The first rule of meal preparation should be using what needs to be used up first. By devising ways to use up the least fresh food and or leftovers first, the meal preparer is forced to be flexible and creative. For this very reason, when I was a chef in commercial restaurants my favorite thing to do was to create the "Daily Special". In most restaurants the daily special is created from

whatever needs to be used up first and it is more challenging than preparing regular menu items.

Changing Our Diet…

It is worth repeating that we are more addicted to the foods we love and our poor eating habits than any "drug addict" is to the most dangerous drugs. Again, what your mind can conceive, you can achieve—meaning that once you grasp and accept the concept that you are what you eat and food is your best medicine, you can be open to change.

I suspect that nearly everyone who is reading this book has probably been consuming meat and dairy products most of their lives. If this is true for you, just let me say to you that this was also true for me. I did not decide to give it all up overnight. In fact, I went through various periods in my life either with or without meat and dairy. Since my cancer, however, I never went back to my earliest high rate of consumption and I have continued to restrict certain animal foods either partially or entirely from my diet while occasionally falling off the wagon—this pertained to sugary and processed foods too.

It has been interesting to me to observe in myself and my wife, Rose, the effects of these dietary changes. When consuming meat, for example, after abstaining for a while, I would feel heavy and weighed down while my body was still digesting for longer periods of time. Rose, often complained of nasal and sinus congestion soon after we indulged ourselves with a little cheese. After some initial cleansing and adjustments in your own diets, you too, will begin to notice how certain foods affect your overall well-being. An intensive cleansing program and/or dietary changes kept to over a period of time will definitely reprogram your dietary palette and food cravings. Once you have achieved this, why go through the self sacrifice of a cleansing program and then re-contaminate yourself with unhealthy food?

But, if you are not already convinced of the benefits of a cleaner and more alkaline diet, you will eventual learn from your own experiences when diligently playing detective and making committed changes along the way.

So, whether you decide that it is better for you to drastically alter your diet right away or to do it gradually, I encourage you to get started. Each step is a positive step, especially if it affects other members of your family, as well. Today, I am convinced of the safety and health benefits of a purely vegan diet, and Rose and I intend to stick to it as best we can throughout our travels. If your health is in crisis, I urge you to do the same. If you are feeling well but want to head off a future crisis, then begin to strive each day to incorporate healthier meals into your menu planning. For those of you not taking the extreme, higher road to healthful dining, I am offering the following food planning advice. Please consider and then practice these rules:

1. Think of a plate of food as a pie and section it into fourths.
2. One fourth should be a fresh, raw salad.
3. One fourth can be more salad or a cooked vegetable(s).
4. One fourth can be a starch like potato, rice, pasta, or tortillas.
5. One fourth can be a protein like beans, seeds and nuts.
6. Animal protein: Only one meal per day and take 2 Pancreatin ½ hour before eating.

Eggs must be fertile from free range hens not feed fed.

Meat should be from the grass grazing animals, lovingly killed by slitting throat and allowed to bleed to death then removing all fat and heavily salt meat to draw out blood, then washing off salt and cooking well.

Cheese preferably made from fresh, raw, healthy milk by separating curds from whey.

Sardines packed in unsalted water seem to be the safest today

7. Make your breakfast and lunch your largest meals.
8. Have a very light supper 12 hours or more before your next day's breakfast so that you fast these 12 hours every day except for water.
9. Chew all food to mush before swallowing and drink only between meals.

Eggs, meat, dairy and fish are not to be eaten by people with cancer or illness

I must confess that eggs and cheese and bread were always my favorite foods. Any combination of the three would do or even individually. In my youth, movies would occasionally depict a criminal soon to be executed given a last meal of anything desired. Usually the meal in the movies was a big steak. I always said my last meal choice would be a cheese omelet perhaps with onions, jalapeños, grilled bread and hash browned potatoes. Giving up good eggs and cheese is a sacrifice I have chosen to make to preserve my health. Giving up meat is easier when I think of not eating corpses.

Rose's healthful recipes...

Finally, in this section, Rose wanted to include a few user-friendly and good-tasting recipes. Mostly we tend to improvise and create with what needs to be used up or what is readily available. When it comes to baking, however, it is necessary to be more precise. We decided to only include a few basic ideas here and let you be the ultimate creator. I never did like following a recipe—if you haven't got exactly what it calls for, then what? You need to learn to substitute and experiment. However, having a few good references on hand may help to give you some novel ideas when you find yourself in the doldrums. When first learning to cook more healthfully, Rose's favorite cooking magazine was *Vegetarian Times.* Whatever turns out to be your favorite recipe book or resource, try not to become too dependent on it.

ROSE'S GARDEN VEGETABLE SALAD

Ingredients:

Chopped Onion (red adds more color)
Finely chopped clove of garlic (optional)
Chopped Tomato
Chopped Green Pepper
Diced Cucumber or Zucchini
Diced Yellow Squash
Chopped Celery or Chinese Bok-Choy
Shredded Carrot
Shredded Cabbage ($^1/_3$–$^1/_2$ total volume)

Use any or all of the above or anything else in season you can think of, such as chow-chow which can be shredded raw. Combine lots of color and texture for a nutritious and delicious garden salad.

Dressing:

Add a pinch or two of sea salt (Real Salt)
Juice of a lime
Extra virgin olive oil
Marie's hot sauce (I prefer the green) – optional

Toss and Serve

Make a large bowl since this will keep in Tupperware in the refrigerator a few days. Another added option when on a regular diet is to throw in some raisins (always better the next day) or chopped apple unless the combination gives you indigestion.

GRATED BEET SALAD

Fresh Grated Beets
Diced Cucumber
Chopped Onion
Add
Fresh squeezed lime juice
A pinch or two of sea salt
Just enough extra virgin olive oil to moisten

Mix and Serve

Grated Beet salad is an easy, raw addition to any meal that also dresses up any plate.

WHOLESOME CHEWY CARROT COOKIES

2 cups whole wheat flour
2 teaspoons baking powder
¼ teaspoon sea salt
2 cups rolled oats
½ cup or more sunflower seeds
1 cup chopped walnuts
½ cup or more raisins
2 cups shredded *carrot
1 cup honey
1 cup extra virgin olive oil
Grated rind of 2 limes

Preheat oven to 375 F.
Combine flour, baking powder, salt and oats, and mix well.
Stir in seeds, nuts, raisins, carrots and lime rind.
Beat together oil and honey.
Stir into flour mixture until well moistened.
Drop by well-rounded teaspoonfuls onto an oiled baking sheet, pat and compress slightly till held together.
Bake for 10-12 minutes until lightly colored. Let sit one minute on sheet, and then transfer to a rack to cool.
Recipe makes about 40 cookies.

*If you are low on carrots, add some zucchini—Remember, don't be afraid to experiment.

Bon Appetite!

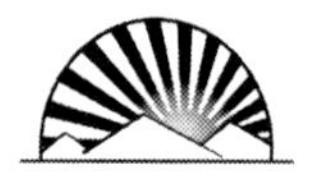

Chapter Six: **How to Eliminate Stress**

Stress is a modern buzz word. It has been blamed for everything and perhaps rightly so. Stress is usually defined as, "a state of extreme difficulty, pressure or strain". However, also consider that some stress can be beneficial. If we never exert or stress our muscles we will become soft and flabby. If we are never pressured to think and act quickly we will become unprepared for emergencies. What brings on harmful stress varies from person to person and situation to situation. But, in my opinion, there are some common threads. They are poor diet, lack of exercise, financial worries and lack of faith in God. In this chapter, we will discuss exercise and financial worries. Since you have already come this far, perhaps you are already changing your diet and are renewing your relationship with our Heavenly Father.

Exercise—Use it or lose it...

In today's modern, urban society most people awake from the bed, move to a chair or couch and then with very short walks in between go from couch to car to chair and back to bed. This is what we call a sedentary lifestyle. Contrast this with life in rural society. You might awake from the bed at dawn and have chores before breakfast like feeding animals, checking the gardens or walking the fence line. Most of the day is spent outside until dusk at various tasks with food breaks in between. Perhaps you should move to the country? If not, you must find a way to get off your butt in the city.

A sedentary lifestyle causes obesity and toxicity. Regular exertion burns fat and causes better immunity, improved circulation, retention of calcium, better muscle tone, better function of heart and lungs, and much less fatigue. I used the word exertion instead of exercise above because in order to see results from exercise you must exert yourself enough to raise your pulse rate and breathing to break and maintain a sweat for several minutes each day. This raises your basic metabolic rate that requires more fuel to convert to energy. If you are not eating quick-energy food, the body begins to burn either what it has too much of, or what it needs least, or both. This is usually the excess fat but it could be tumors or other diseased tissue as well. Solid fat cells are converted into liquid fat called lipids to provide energy by combustion. Picture a train progressing from standing still to slowly gaining speed and needing more fuel as the demand increases until it comes to a hill and then it really has to burn more fuel. Exercise increases the burning of fuel. Sweating cleanses the body of toxins.

Let me paint another word picture for you. You have an older model car. It only gets driven once a week to the grocery store and once a week to church and at a slow speed. Because you put very few miles on your car each year, you do not spend very much money on tune ups, oil changes and fuel additives. One day on the way to town, you are about to cross a railroad crossing when you see the train coming. "I can make it across", you say and step on the gas to pick up speed and the car sputters, backfires and stalls right on the track. The end of that story I will leave to your imagination, but you can clearly see that fitness and maintenance pay off. If you suddenly need your body to perform in order to prevent an accident, can it?

Dr. Herbert M. Shelton, an authority on natural healing and practitioner of Natural Hygiene, wrote in his book

Exercise! "Exercise may be truly considered the most important vital tonic of the body. If it is wholly neglected, the body will become weak, and all its physical powers will be diminished; but regularly and properly indulged in, the whole system will be strengthened and invigorated."

The simplest form of exercise is to stand up and walk. Why are the simplest things in life sometimes the most difficult? All you really need is a good, supportive pair of walking shoes and a pleasant stretch of real estate away from traffic to practice your stride. Whatever the form of exercise you choose, your goals should be to increase flexibility and endurance. Building tightness and bulk may look good to some but it is not beneficial for you in the long term. Stretching and holding the stretch for at least thirty seconds increases flexibility. Endurance comes from exerting yourself long enough to sweat. The simplest stretch that I use is to bend from the waist keeping my knees straight and letting my arms and hands hang down until I touch the floor. I hold this for at least thirty seconds then very slowly raise my arms up over head and stretch backwards. I push against a post in our bedroom or living room when upright arching my back and reaching upward.

Another key to beneficial exercise is to work at strengthening the legs, which function as your second heart. Walking or rebounding on a mini-trampoline to me is the best for this. Although we have no financial interest in recommending it, we really love our Needak® rebounder with the support bar. The benefits of rebounding are too numerous for me to go into here. Linda Brooks, in her book, *Rebounding to Better Health*, covers it all. Children seem to instinctively know that bouncing must be good for them and bounce on beds and furniture whenever given the chance. Besides being fun, what I especially like is the fact that rebounding is easy and convenient for all ages; a reasonable investment; puts a positive stress on each cell of the body without stressing your joints; and in addition to increasing our cardiovascular circulation, it stimulates our lymphatic system which flushes toxins and waste products out of the body. So, check Needak® out, they are the best.

You do not have to belong to a fancy health club or buy expensive home equipment to exercise. Small choices in our daily routine can make a big difference. Most people live on one floor. If they live above the ground floor, they take the elevator. We designed our homes here to be eight feet off the ground not only for better air circulation and less dampness but also to force us to go up and down stairs many times each day, great for the legs, heart and lungs.

By incorporating deep or diaphragmatic breathing into your exercise, you receive the most benefit and by doing it often enough you will impregnate this into the memory bank of your autonomic nervous system and it will eventually become an automatic part of your subconscious or involuntary functions.

Remember that muscles are mostly designed to be antagonistic. One set of muscles work against the other to produce balance—the flexors work against the extensors and the biceps work against the triceps, etc. Two very important sets of antagonistic muscles are our abdominal and low back muscles. Whenever you see a person with a sagging gut you can bet that they have low back problems. The lower back and spine are supported by the tone of both the front (abdominal) and rear (low back) muscle groups. When the front is weak the back is called upon to make up the imbalance resulting in strain and pain. Of course the lesson here is to get in shape. Rid yourself of any excess load you are carrying around like the bag of cement I talked about—creating a physical imbalance (page 58). Colon cleansing, diet change, rebounding and walking will produce a new you.

Years ago, when membership status meant something to me, I joined a fancy health club. I must admit that there was a signing bonus of a free trip to Las Vegas that enticed me most. When I sweat now—either when working outdoors or from the natural air (without air-conditioning) inside—I remember how much I paid each month for the privilege of sweating at a fancy club. You do not need costly clubs or equipment to tone up or sweat. Just do it!

More ideas for exercise:

- Give away your weed eater and buy a machete and 3 sided file to keep it sharp. I am still amazed what one person can do with a machete once you get the rhythm down.
- Do not jog or run on hard pavement and especially not alongside vehicle traffic where you breathe exhaust fumes.
- Create your own walking trail on your land or go to a quiet street or park to walk.
- Do as much of your own maintenance and repair as you can.

A Reawakening and Re-dedication...

It is interesting to me and perhaps to you also that even small events seem to happen for a reason. When we relocated from the U.S. to Belize, we needed to cut our possessions "to the bone" because of the high cost of shipping, duty and tax. Rose and I owned many books. My dream was always to have my own library room. I love books but here in Belize they mold with age. We carefully sifted through our beloved books and shipped only the best representation or two on many subjects.

When we began researching and refreshing our information for this book, we reread many of our books. One in particular stands out among many and that is the book *Exercise* by Dr. Herbert M. Shelton from whom I previously quoted. In my opinion, this is the definitive book on the subject and it has inspired me to rethink my posture and exercise program to strengthen myself more. The chapter on hernia correction has inspired me to strengthen myself rather than resort to surgery. A strong body is needed to maintain external and internal posture not only of muscles, but position of internal organs. Dr. Shelton stresses this point throughout his book. Muscle building is not solely for the sake of appearances. More importantly, it is to enable all of our organs and systems to function properly. Get with it and get in shape, for the love of God!

Keeping your mind fit is equally as important as keeping the rest of you fit. Our brain uses 65% of our body's nutrition so a proper diet is as important as is exercising our brain. Brain cells die off and need to be replaced. Inactivity breeds stagnation. Learn something new every day. Awake like a child eager to seize the day and experience whatever comes along. Read and discuss ideas and feelings with others. Continue to marvel and learn, exercise the mind by taking up new challenges, whether it is knitting or the rebuilding of a clock—whatever turns you on and stimulates your creativity in order to keep building new brain cells. Keeping exposure to a minimum, the Internet can provide information on most any subject if you use it wisely. Better yet, get up, get out and go to a library. Teach the young what you know and invite their questions. Develop interest in what the young are thinking and doing.

Learning to cope financially…

In my senior year at Podiatry College, we had a course called "Medical Economics". It was scheduled only one day each week for two hours. The teacher was a noted Podiatrist, Dr. E., who drove three hours each way from another city. Dr. E. was very well known on the lecture/convention circuit not only for his seminars but also for his very large, successful private practice. It was said that his office saw 60–80 patients daily, run by a very large staff of assistants, and that his income was in the six figures—this was back in the early 60s.

My first day in Medical Economics class, Dr. E. arrived fifteen minutes late, looking rather florid and portly in his hand-tailored sharkskin suit, silk tie and shirt and patent leather loafers. He strode to the blackboard and wrote, "#1. Establish financial stability". He then proceeded to spend the remainder of the two hours talking on why we should not be in debt. This was very reassuring for a senior student praying for a friendly bank to help him get started. As it turned out, I was drawn to open my practice in Dallas because of the friendly banking policy towards new Podiatrists who were needed at the time. Easy credit got me into financial pressures many times since then until I learned the lesson I had ignored way back from Dr. E.

Let me describe another personal scenario and see if you can relate to it. When I was growing up I had an uncle who was a stock broker. Most of our family began buying stocks because of his advice. I would often visit him at the brokerage offices where he worked on my way home from high school, since they were near my bus connection. How impressed I was by the ticker tape and the "big board", brokers talking to clients on the phone and in person as they wrote orders for buying or selling many shares of stock. I saved enough to buy $100 of stock in a company advised by my uncle. I was hooked. Every day I would look for my stock in the newspaper. I made a chart and graphed each up and down. My heart would ache when the stock went down and leap when it went up. I sold that stock within two years just before it went way up.

Coincidentally, the very stock I invested in as a youth forms the basis of an object lesson in corporate greed. Until the 1950s, electric streetcars or "trolley cars" were the method of public transportation in most cities. They ran on steel wheels on rails imbedded in cobblestone streets which were virtually indestructible. The power came from electric overhead wires connected to the streetcar by a "trolley" or long connecting rod. Each end of the trolley car had controls for the conductor who switched ends to return the way he had come. He also had to disconnect the rear trolley rod and connect the front one. Streetcars were simple and non-polluting.

Then General Motors Corp founded a subsidiary called National City Line. This was the new stock my uncle advised me to buy for my $100 investment. GMC was building new, modern, air-conditioned, diesel engine buses. They were convincing city managers to change from the old-fashioned streetcars to new diesel buses and to tear up all the bumpy cobblestone streets, tracks and all and re-pave with smooth black tar. I always say that if you want to know the truth then follow the money trail. Who benefited from this changeover, certainly GMC and the oil companies and probably some city managers as well? The public has not benefited from the diesel fumes or the constant re-paving of streets. Today cities are either converting back to electric buses or wishing they could. That example of corporate manipulation and marketing is penny ante compared to the global greed of today.

Later as an adult, when I was in private practice, I began buying and charting stocks on borrowed money. The stresses of the daily ups and downs were now magnified compared to my experience as a youth. Monthly payments eventually brought on illness.

Are you invested in the stock market? It took me a long time to break the gambling addiction of the stock market. I finally came to the conclusion that it is an insiders game and if you do not have the insider's information, you had better be a huge player that can cause small ups and downs by your buying and selling. The instant I was completely out of the stock market, a tremendous weight fell from my shoulders.

Somewhere in the past, our generation was heavily marketed to "Buy American" and we still are today. This philosophy is great for corporations to lure money and for brokers who make money when you buy or sell. Investing in someone else to make money for you has become a dangerous way of life unless you really know and trust that person or company intimately. "Investing" has become a national lifestyle whether it is in stocks, bonds, commodities or various other schemes for which we ourselves do not physically participate other than signing documents.

We should be investing extra money either in ourselves or someone close to us whom we love and trust. Just think of all the creativity that could be unleashed if we used our investment money to improve our own business or help a younger relative start out. When I was on the board of directors of the Fayetteville Farmer's Market there was much discussion about what to do with the thousands of dollars in local bank accounts accumulated over many years. Another vendor urged the board to let a friend who was an investment counselor make a presentation. A date was set and the counselor showed us with charts and graphs how she would invest and diversify our one hundred thousand plus dollars. After she left, I urged the board to reject stock investment and invest in making the market better. The stock idea got tabled indefinitely and individual farmers told me how they were switching personal investments from stocks to themselves.

Divest yourself of unnecessary expense...

In these troubling times of financial uncertainty, re-evaluation is a must if you are stressed over money. Downsizing is the answer. Many years ago I realized that if I did not downsize my life to a point where I could exist on a minimum of income with no debt, my future would be stressful. Let me take you through the steps I took to where I am today.

First you must eliminate monthly payments except for the absolute essentials. You are not much good to yourself or anyone else unless you have health and vitality. If you have made a commitment to regain and maintain your health, then you should have begun to realize that your dependence on doctors, pharmacies and medical insurance is lessening. Once you have become empowered with the God-given ability to heal yourself then why have medical insurance at all? We have not paid one penny into the insurance lottery game for decades. We need hospitals and doctors to put us back together if we are injured but we do not need them to keep us healthy. If you must buy insurance, buy accident or catastrophic coverage.

Another financial trap is your home. If you are making payments to rent or buy a home, then a priority is to eliminate home payments. The best advice I can give you at this time is to liquidate as much as you can, take your losses and move somewhere you can afford to live easily. Find a small rural community where you can buy very reasonably or better yet build your own home with no permit or zoning restrictions and low taxes. Ground yourself in a local church and discover what real neighbors are all about. When you liquidate, you must put aside enough to cover your bare living expenses for one or two years, relocation expenses, home building or buying costs and enough to start a small business. Wow! You've got to be kidding, you say? I'm not kidding! If you are under financial stress, you must make drastic long term changes.

Let me back up and give you some more insights on the above statements. When we first moved to this charming third-world country of Belize, I was shocked to hear the Prime Minister say to a high school graduating class, "Do not look for a job, start a business". He probably said that because there are not enough businesses to create jobs. However, he was 100% right in my opinion. When you own your own business in the USA you have automatically created your own personal tax shelter just like the "big boys". You are eligible for all the incentives, tax credits, deductions and "loopholes" that enable the rich to pay very little tax on what they actually earn. You can still have a job and own a small business and use the expenses and losses of that small business to offset the taxes you have deducted from your pay check each week. Big business has experts peruse the tax rules each year to find ways to take advantage of tax loopholes. You can do the same with a small business. Invest in yourself.

If we take a backward look at history, we find that taxes were imposed by governments as a temporary measure to finance extra expenditures such as war. When the war was over, the taxes were supposed to be done away with. Taxes were originally levied on corporations not individuals. Now, corporations pay far less taxes per dollar of income than individuals who bear most of the burden.

When I first decided to "go back to the land", there was no clear plan except a vision to go to rural Arkansas. I had left all assets behind and set out with all I owned in a used, orange VW pop-top van. Never had I felt so free then or since. There is a great lifting of weight when you divest yourself of all possessions. I can imagine the stress free existence of a monk, can you? That van and I had great adventures together. Because I had a "mobile home", I was invited to stay at many farms and private retreats after meeting new friends. By the time my mother joined me, I had learned enough to risk buying a small house in a small town. We later sold that small house and our bakery, which gave us enough for me to build our own hexagonal, post and beam home on the community farm where we lived prior to moving here to Belize in 2005. Building your own home with your own hands and help from some friends and eating food from your own garden is a blessing I pray you may one day receive as I have. Here in Belize we were able to buy tropical hardwood houses, custom built by the Mennonites and delivered to our home site well within our relocation budget. We did the interior and utility work ourselves along with local help.

Cultivating new options...

The best start up business I could think of right now would be a local market gardener. Become a miniature farmer and grow healthy vegetables in your home garden for your local community. The demand for clean, local produce is growing (pun intended). I will discuss this issue again in the chapter on agriculture and again in the last chapter because it is a seed that needs to be planted many times until many begin to sprout new rural farm communities. If your resources are slim, then pool and share resources with several other families so that you have enough to buy or rent enough land so that each family has about six acres. Now you have a mini-farm. You can share equipment with your neighbors and rotate crops among you. This is already happening so you better ride this new economic wave.

Your home can be your business and part of it can be deducted. A farm also has more tax benefits than the average business. There are many opportunities all around us if we do not limit our thinking. First of all, dare to dream like a small child and imagine what you would do if you could do anything you wanted? If you find something that you can be good at and it serves others with love, your business will be a success. But don't forget the very small details which determine success or failure and be willing to work.

Keep your monthly fixed overhead low. We have become miserly about using electricity and driving. We own one four-cylinder pickup and keep it carefully maintained. At this writing, gas here in Belize is $4.50/gal US. We invested in an LP gas conversion kit and when gas goes to $5.00 US, we run on butane at almost half the price. The mileage is a little less on LP. Since giving up TV and the high cost of cable, we now have more time for conversation. We watch selected DVDs and pre-recorded special programs from when we did have TV.

Are you starting to get the idea? Whatever your financial stress, it can be removed if you are willing to change. If you live in a city, begin to think seriously about relocating to the country. With the advent of the Internet, we can search out anything anywhere and even via satellite zoom in for an actual look. Even before the recent financial crisis, there have been thousands of rural properties taken over by lending institutions. This number has recently multiplied and now lending institutions are holding rural properties that they are willing to wheel and deal on. If a property has been vacant for a long time, you may be able to create a very favorable arrangement with the lender.

If you live in a city and there is no way you are capable of relocating to the country, then you really have got to become creative in your financial stress-free thinking. Perhaps you need to move to a less expensive neighborhood. Another possibility is to unite neighbors in your own neighborhood to work together to achieve a common goal, creating a win-win situation. Creating a neighborhood garden is an excellent way to begin. It could be on vacant land, on rooftops, or in small plots and containers. Suburbs often have housing developments where the backyards face each other creating a contiguous park. What a great place this would be for a community or block garden. Also think about collecting your own water off of your roof not only for gardening, but for your own use as well—best to filter, especially well, before drinking.

Finally the last financial investment advice I am going to give you is from Eccl. 11:1, "Cast thy bread upon the waters: for thou shalt find it after many days". There is no doubt in my mind that the more you give in service to the Lord by serving others and/or by tithing, in some way you will be repaid many times over.

Reversal of current trends...

I feel, once again, like a voice in the wilderness crying out—but no one pays any attention.

When I reflect on our present-day societies compared to how life was in early Bible times, the most startling revelation is where we have been led—like the rats following the "Pied Piper of Hamlin" to their doom. By ignoring basic principles from God and following "free choice", most societies have adopted "democracy" and a "free market" economy. What does this mean? A democratic society elects people to govern them and create laws supposedly for the well-being of the voters. There is a separation of Church and State. A "free market" economy is based upon the principle of "capitalism", which is, in my opinion, "to turn something to ones own advantage". The "laws of supply and demand" control prices and the aim is to "buy low and sell high". Is modern capitalistic, democratic society anything like God intended us to live our lives? I think not.

The Bible teaches us that interest should be charged to strangers and that should never exceed ten-percent. Every fiftieth year was to be declared a "year of jubilee" when all debts would be abolished and "...ye shall return every man unto his possession, and ye shall return every man unto his family" (Lev. 25:10). Thus, the land could not be alienated forever. This law also pertains to the keeping of Sabbaths including the resting of land in seven year cycles.

How different life is today when most businesses double their investments and when most farmers are more concerned with increasing their yields per acre than nurturing the land for future generations; when manufacturers are more concerned with increasing productivity by lowering the cost of labor; and when governments have become the private club of special wealthy corporations.

There is only one way you can help to change this downward spiral and escape being led to the river to drown by the pied piper of greed and that is to change yourself first. Be the one to set yourself apart and be an example that others would want to follow—an example that is peace loving and law abiding, considerate of your fellow man and honoring of God.

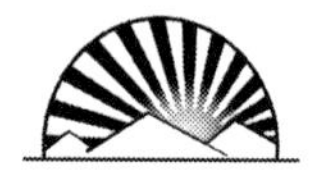

Chapter Seven: **Agriculture, Ecology and You**

The agriculture discussed in this chapter is not what is currently taught in mainstream colleges. It is about learning how to tune in to the land around you and nurture it and sustain it for future generations, not bending it to your will. We can only begin to arouse first your curiosity and then your passion for growing healthy food. Astute observation of your land over several seasons and years will teach you the best lessons.

As you become more in tune with the health of your own body, it usually follows that you become more aware of the health of your immediate environment either at home or at work. Probably you become most aware of the food you eat several times a day and how that food affects your health. When you reach the consciousness where you become concerned about where your food comes from and how it was grown, then you are at the intersection of three forks in your road. You can continue on the road straight ahead which is buying your food at the store and trust the labeling. Or you can choose the road to the left, which is seeking out local growers directly at the farm or at farmers' markets. The road to the right takes you to growing your own food in a manner that sustains the earth.

Of course you know already what is coming since I have chosen the road to the right many years ago and I am now calling you to follow. When you become concerned about what you feed yourself, as well as others, then you need to return to the land. God made Adam and Eve caretakers or stewards of the Garden of Eden. He did not give them ownership. The land wherever it is belongs to God, not to humanity. It is humanity's responsibility to be a caretaker and good steward of Gods' land. Does that mean we should rape it of anything saleable and then milk it for every cent it will produce without regard for God or future generations? You cannot worship two gods. If you care more about increasing yields of bushels per acre than you do about the health of the land, then you are serving money not God. There is a vital chain linked between God, the earth, our food and us. To not have respect for one link in this chain is to not have respect for every link as they are inseparable. The ideas discussed in this small chapter are only meant to inspire you to learn more and use them as the seeds of change.

A new peaceful revolution

Most of you are not old enough to remember the Chinese Communist Revolution led by Chairman Mao Tse Tung. There were many brutal methods used to get rid of the opposition, mostly death. The main mission was to take from the hands of the greedy and give to the hands of the needy. People in cities were forced to go and work on the land. In essence it was an agricultural revolution. People began to appreciate and nurture the land where their food came from. The result was a nation of small farmers living in rural communities without a dramatic hierarchy of wealth and class. Today, now that capitalism has crept in, large corporate agriculture and food production, based on the US model, has returned to China.

What we need in the capitalistic countries in this time of crisis is the break up of large agro-business (corporate farming) and the introduction of incentives for people without work to return to small family farming. This may take place over time rather than a sudden change. Can you imagine what an evolution that would be? The small Christian family farm was and should be the backbone of any society. Land that is nurtured according to biblical principles—not milked for every cent—is what will restore not only the health of the soil but also our health as well. More incentives and subsidies are needed for families to grow our food—not multi-national agro-business. I will discuss more on what moral values are instilled by family farm life in Chapter Nine.

Hundreds of thousands of acres are not being farmed that could be revived to become productive using sustainable methods—not chemical means of rescue from the environment. We need to give people the motivation to return to small family farming instead of underwriting corporate America, which has been government policy for too long. However, we should not become too dependent on government for anything except our national defense. While writing this chapter, it was a joy to read an article in USA Today about young families and singles returning to the land and practicing small scale sustainable mini-farming on 6–7 acres. That article confirmed and implied that this may be the beginning of a new economic wave, a peaceful revolution.

The seven acre mini-farm

Right now and today I am challenging you and your relatives and friends to gather your resources and head for the country. But first do some homework. The best place for information that I know about is the National Sustainable Agriculture Information Service—known as ATTRA—whose website is www.attra.ncat.org/ (ATTRA was formerly known as the "Appropriate Technology Transfer for Rural Areas" project.). Located in Fayetteville, Arkansas, ATTRA is the information arm of NCAT—

National Center for Appropriate Technology. They are the "gurus" of sustainable agriculture. Subscribe to their free online newsletters. With a seven-acre farm, you could have one acre for residence and outbuildings and six acres for agriculture. Divide these acres into as many plots as you wish, but always keep a rotation of one acre fallow each year after planting a cover crop such as fava beans. With adjoining seven-acre farms belonging to family or friends, you can share equipment and plan a rotation and marketing of non-conflicting produce. I discussed the financial and tax benefits of this previously.

A word of caution is water. Be assured that you will have enough available water to grow what you want to grow. Is there enough annual rainfall and how is it distributed throughout an average year? Are there roofs for collecting rainwater in cisterns? Are there accessible wells, ponds, creeks, rivers or lakes nearby to tap as a water source? Without water, you cannot grow.

Start by beginning to build good soil...

Don't be overwhelmed! Whether you have one-tenth acre or seven acres or more, the principles are the same. First of all start a compost pile. A compost pile is a pile of any organic matter that will decay and rot. Compost is your best fertilizer. Manures and animal wastes can be composted with plant material, but may attract more animal scavengers and flies and may need to be screened. Selecting a site is important. I prefer a covered metal, pole shed roof with half walls of roofing on three sides leaving the front open for access but blocked from animal access with 24-inch high, welded wire. A large composting area needs to be accessible to a front end loader (see illustration). Divide the inside space into two sections with a half wall. The more growing plots you have, the more compost you will need, so build your compost shed proportionately. One side of the compost bin is active while the other side is inactive while covered with a tarp and allowed to cook. In climates with a winter season, we rotated bins every year. In the sub-tropical climate, where we are now, things break down faster and we are on a six month rotation. We use a base of whatever we can get free or low cost such as straw or hardwood sawdust. I try to avoid hay with seed heads that will eventually sprout grass in your growing beds. We spread the compost from the inactive side on our growing beds when we are ready to rest our active side. Each day we empty our compost bucket in the kitchen into a hole dug in the active bin and we also empty our porta-potty buckets at the same time. We then cover over the hole and move the ever present shovel to a new digging place for next time.

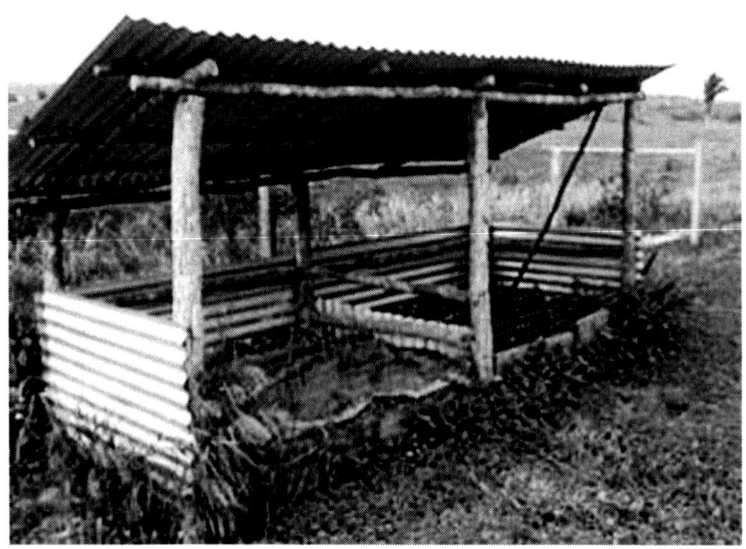

Compost Bins

I must comment briefly at this point that our flush and forget toilet society epitomizes lack of responsibility. First of all, if you are health conscious, then it is important to not only be careful about what you put into you, but also you need to be more conscious about what comes out of you. Knowing what is coming out of you is especially important during a cleansing. The resulting manure then becomes a valuable fertilizer after being broken down by composting—a process of 6-12 months, depending on climate. If you live in the city, we advise using a five-gallon plastic bucket with a little citrus degreaser and water in the bottom to catch your bowel movements and urine, for your personal inspection as well as for gardening. Urban composting can be done in a plastic barrel.

Let's have a brief discussion about topsoil. Topsoil is the top 3–6 inches of your land. I have heard about land where the rich topsoil was more than a foot deep, but have only lived on marginal land after it had been mostly logged off. Even on small plots, soil varies. If you are fortunate enough to have good topsoil, you can build your garden bed. Plan a four-foot wide bed with a walkway around it. Move soil from the walkway areas into the garden area to create a raised bed. What you need to nurture is the top 3–6 inches. If you have poor or no topsoil then you have to create the growing material that will comprise your bed. This can be done by redistributing extra soil on your own land or bringing in dirt, sand, peat moss and other ingredients from off your land and creating your own starting mixture which should improve every year if nurtured.

Compost, mulches and green manures are the sustainable ways to enrich your soil without resorting to agro-chemicals. Mulches are coverings for your growing beds that retain moisture, prevent soil erosion, break down to provide nutrients, and suppress weeds. The soil in your growing area, if possible, should never be exposed and naked. The mulch can be anything from the residue of the recently harvested crop to a layer of alfalfa hay, which I used to like best when I could buy it fairly reasonably. Green manures or cover crops are grown usually between crops to re-enrich the soil and to choke out weeds. There are many options for cover crops. I like beans which bring nitrogen into the soil and particularly fava beans or cow peas. Cowpeas are cheap and grow fast. Fava beans are more expensive and slower to grow but produce an enormous mass of vegetation to enrich your soil. We chop beans down with a machete when ½ of them are in blossom, wait about a week and then plant thru the mulch or sometimes lightly cultivate with a 3-inch hand tine tool. This manner of planting without tilling the field is called "no till". With it, the soil always has a covering. That is why the practice of no-till has become popular with sustainable farmers.

Working with the soil...

Now, where to begin your growing? If you have space then raised beds are the way to go. Raised beds drain quicker and better define your growing space from the walkways in between. If you have a large operation and are using mechanized equipment, you can form raised beds between the wheel widths of your tractor. However, I urge you to stay small enough to work your mini farm with mostly non-motorized tools. For hand work, a four-foot-wide bed works best as it enables someone to reach halfway from both sides without stepping into the bed. Once formed, avoid walking on your beds which will compact the soil.

You can define the borders of your beds several ways. My favorite, when funds are available, is to purchase rough sawn 2x6 hardwood lumbers, as reasonably as possible, by buying old boards or too poor quality for construction. No treated lumber can be used on your land if you are truly health conscious. We then cut off two 4-foot pieces for each end of the bed and begin forming the sides by connecting boards with an interior splice. We drill and screw everything together. Before adding the soil you may want to either chop all vegetation removing roots, put down a sheet of thin plastic or cardboard which will smother undergrowth and slowly break down. After the soil is added and leveled out up to the edges of the boards six inches

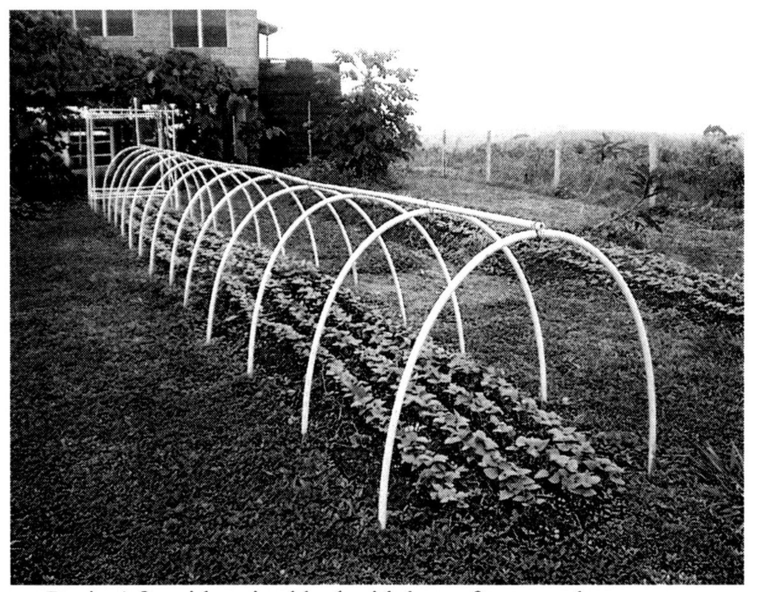

Basic 4 ft. wide raised bed with hoop frame and cover crop

deep, I like to hammer an 18-inch piece of rebar one foot into the ground every three feet against the outside leaving six inches above ground. We then create a hoop over the bed with a ¾-inch PVC pipe cut seven feet long and slipped over the six-inch of rebar from side to side. To support and space your hoops secure a straight piece of pipe to the top outside of the hoop with twist ties or cable ties. Connect additional lengths by joining but not gluing. This framework can serve multiple purposes for shade cloth, row cover, or poly in colder weather. You can certainly have great raised beds without the above framework by defining your walkways either by mowing and edging and/or the use of gravel, sawdust, straw or whatever you wish.

Start out with a cover crop of beans then begin planting. Do not till, but occasional hand cultivation with a 3– to 6-inch three-tine cultivator is acceptable. Rotate your crops so that you do not plant the same crop in the same bed every time. Keep some beds fallow with a cover crop every year and rotate. Get involved with your local farmer's market or create one. Encourage people to come directly to your farm to buy. A new trend is on-the-farm dining if you are skilled at both growing and cooking.

Start a seed bank…

Good seed is becoming scarce and may not be available at all in the future. Invest in yourself by buying as many varieties and as much quantity as you can afford of: First, heirloom seed which are old, rare, original species then; Second, open pollinated seeds. These seeds will bear heartier and more naturally resistant crops. Learn to save seed from your crops. No hybrid seed or genetically modified seed should be bought. These seeds are bred to require chemical input and seed saved from hybrids will not reproduce the original. Store your seed in an air tight container in your freezer. Important information: when you want to plant some of your seed, remove only that to be sown and spread on a plate or tray in natural light for two weeks. The explanation for this is that when the seeds are frozen they become dormant and allowing them to gradually revive before planting will insure that your germination will be near 100 percent.

When first beginning to grow, try small plots of a wide variety of your seed and see what likes to grow where. Although large scale row cropping has become the method used in commercial agriculture these days, you will never see mono-culture plots in nature. Man has been intent on subduing nature rather than trying to work with it in harmony. I have become less fanatical about weeds in my growing beds because many of them have medicinal uses. Allow native plants to come up wherever they will and then carefully inspect them and check them out in herbal remedy books. You can always chop them down for mulch if they seem to have no apparent use. Some beds we have let go entirely native to species that have healing properties.

More of my thoughts on "weeds"...

I have been doing a lot of gardening lately and so, naturally, weeds have been on my mind as well as in my garden. As a very small child, I remember crawling on the grass of our small backyard and being enthralled with the little yellow flowers that bloomed there in the spring. However, much to my amazement, no one wanted dandelions in their grass and much time and energy was spent by adults in prying them up with a two-pronged tool. Today, they more often use the latest lawn and garden weed killer instead.

During my infancy and adolescence, we lived in a neighborhood of modest one and two family homes. Immediately next door on one side of us was a ninety-six year old lady Mrs. Ashley, and her spinster daughter. I distinctly remember that Mrs. Ashley asked everyone in the neighborhood that she knew to save the dandelions for her.

With these "weeds", she made tea, soup and even wine. Mrs. Ashley obviously knew something that we didn't.

When I revolted against organized medicine and began my quest to relearn natural healing, one of my goals was to become an organic farmer. I began to read books and the first book I read was called *Secrets of the Soil*. The first statement that jumped out at me in this book was, "a weed is a plant that you do not know yet". Much later, when I was an apprentice to a master organic farmer, I was assigned the lowly job of weeding his vegetable gardens.

During my long hours of toiling with a hoe in hand, my observation showed me that first of all, the weeds had many holes in them from being eaten by insects, much, much more than the veggies we were growing and when the weeds had been removed, the insects began to eat our valued crop with a vengeance. Perhaps the insects knew something that we didn't?

Weeds are a lot like people. We tend to not want to know people who are different from us. But, if we were to really get to know them, we might find that they have much value.

Rose and I were a lot like weeds when we came to Spanish Lookout. We feel blessed that many chose to know us. In this next year and beyond, learn more about the weeds in your neighborhood and may the coming years fill you with the blessings and love of our Lord in His gardens.

What about the bugs?

Usually the first question most people ask when considering chemical free agriculture is, "what do you do about the bugs?" Consider this, no bugs, no life.

If you have a lot of bugs you have a healthy environment unless there is an imbalance of good and bad bugs. If you think your environment is healthy because you have the exterminator spray monthly, you are very misguided. I picture the cartoon of the lady chasing a fly through her house while spraying bug killer, and of course breathing it too.

Chemical pesticides have not always proven to be successful at keeping the "bad" bugs away. Is the effort that also poisons our food worth it when these same bugs adapt and come back with a vengeance, forcing the use of stronger pesticides? Besides, not all insects are undesirable. There is a natural balance occurring all the time, at least, when we don't upset this balance of nature. We need to learn to coexist and to make the extra effort it takes to grow food that will sustain our health and the health of the planet.

Insects provide the main source of food for many birds. Attract more birds to your land and you will have fewer insects. Companion planting of wildflowers attracts beneficial insects to your growing area that prey on insects that attack your crops. And, in my opinion, most important of all—and you have probably never heard this said anywhere—insect bites give you minute doses of whatever germs are in your vicinity thereby stimulating an immune boosting response.

There is an energy field around live plants just as there is around our body. Some call this energy field the "aura" and some can see this aura with their eyes. There are special photographic techniques that can record the energy field. People and plants alike have a brighter, stronger energy field when they are healthy. Insects tune in and sense the health of plants by the energy field and they attack the weak and the sickly first. The stronger your plants are, the fewer the insects that will attack them. How do you make your plants strong? The answer is by building soil fertility. As your soil gets richer from natural additives, your crops will become healthier, stronger and insect resistant, provided you planted the best non-hybrid seed.

Well, if you have followed all the rules of good land management and soil enrichment and still the insects are a problem, let me give you some choices that have worked for me. Remember that you are repelling not killing and so a rotation of repellents on a regular schedule works best until the problem lessens. Consider the following:

1. Daily inspection is essential and hand picking of larger insects, worms etc.
2. Spray with an insecticidal soap/water solution.
3. Dust with diatomaceous earth and or kaolin clay.
4. Spray with a hot pepper wax and water solution
5. Dust with cayenne pepper.
6. Spray with a Neem-water solution.
7. Spray with pyrethrums made from marigolds.
8. Use of row covers as a physical barrier.

A higher tech option might be to suck up the bugs! One Sunday we were reading about John in our Sunday school class and about how he preceded Jesus surviving on just "locusts and wild honey". The concept of insects as food obviously is not a new idea. As for wild honey, that is becoming a scarce item as bees are a dying breed. Some biblical scholars have said that when God sends you locusts, then harvest the locusts as your crop. In many parts of the world, farmers are doing just that instead of using chemical pesticides.

There is a new generation of farm equipment designed to be more earth friendly; one of these is a huge vacuum cleaner that sucks the insects from the row crops and collects the harvest. Insects are the food with the highest percentage of pure protein on our planet. The insects gathered can make the best chicken feed imaginable and some countries even add the insect meal to different products for human consumption. I am planting a seed in someone's mind that to own such a piece of equipment could create not only a profitable business but also it might begin to eliminate the need for pesticides which will bring back some wild honey. I have had the thought that a small rechargeable, car vacuum might work for small gardens?

Farming should be a partnership with God and nature...

Remember, whatever you do to the land will have an effect on you and your neighbors. If you use chemicals they eventually work their way through the soil into your water supply and beyond. This is not only a local problem but extends worldwide. In 2003, I wrote the following article for a local paper:

"***Prairie Grove is our "canary in the mine"***

> Many years ago before the advent of industrialization, primitive mines were dug with hand tools which also cut the stone or timbers to shore up the passageways. Torches—and later, oil lamps—provided light and contributed to the other gases released by the digging, to often badly contaminated air in the deeper recesses of the mine. Legend tells us that song birds in cages, often canaries, were carried with the miners into the mines. This is because in case the air quality could not support the life of the bird, they would know that the lives of the miners were in jeopardy. I also like to think that the song

and sight of the bird surely brought brightness to a very drab and hazardous livelihood.

In 2003, the news media in northwest Arkansas heavily reported about the high incidence of cancer in our neighboring community of Prairie Grove. As I recall, local and state agencies could not discover anything, but a privately hired environmental test revealed unusually high levels of arsenic and/or other toxic chemicals in Prairie Grove's environment. There was some mention that this could be related to the many commercial poultry houses and the litter applied to pastures. There was an immediate cry of "foul" from the poultry sacred cow and Prairie Grove is no better off except for more cancer testing under new rural grants.

Prairie Grove was a recent wake up call that our food supply, our environment and our health are inexorably linked together. The answers for Prairie Grove are not more cancer screenings, surgeries, radiations, chemotherapies or high dollar research but more education on how to change our contamination of our food, air, water and ourselves, which will cure and prevent cancer, lower medical costs, and create environmentally friendly industries.

Recently, a friend came over for fellowship. He told me that the corn crop was ready to harvest, but there were problems this year. Most growers were finding many worms in their corn—another sign of environmental change. The reason for this, he said was due to the heavy rain during the growing season. I suspect, yet, another cause.

Earlier this year we were blessed to have a pair of doves make a nest under one of our buildings. We tried not to disturb their egg sitting process and they seemed to accept our occasional peeking. It seemed that they sat on those eggs an unusually long time, but no baby birds appeared. Then we noticed that they had started another nest under another house. The same thing occurred. No baby birds arrived. They started several more nests, abandoning un-hatched eggs each time until recently, one of our cats picked off one of the doves ending that cycle.

When we first moved to Spanish Lookout we marveled each year when flocks of parrots would fly over our house heading for the corn fields. Every year since then, the flocks have been getting smaller and smaller. Could this be that birds are become fewer and fewer due to eggs not hatching? Much undisputable research has been done worldwide linking the use of herbicides and pesticides to infertility and birth defects in animals and humans.

Birds are our #1 defense against insects that attack our crops—fewer birds mean more worms. Birds are also an indicator of the health of our environment. First it was a decline in our bees. Now it is a decline in our birds. Are we being good caretakers of God's land? Are we leaving it better than we found it? Or are we just "milking" it for every penny we can and not worrying what we are leaving to the next generation?

In an essay "Nature as Measure" by Wendell Berry included in the book, *What Are People For?* Berry writes, "Farming cannot take place except in nature; therefore, if nature does not thrive, farming cannot thrive...If it does not thrive, we cannot thrive. The appropriate measure of farming then is the world's health and our health, and this is inescapably one measure."

Bio-diversity

One of the reasons I moved to the Ozark Mountains of Arkansas in 1983 was to explore the wilderness and identify medicinal plants. Most of the hardwood forest then was in third and fourth generation growth. It was traditional practice among the older land owners to burn the underbrush early in the spring when the surface was dry and while the ground still retained moisture from late snow. One "old timer" told me that after the brush has been burned off several years, then the really old species of plants, trees and bushes begin to come up from seeds long buried.

I urge you to leave plots of ground unattended on your land and observe what comes up. Identify these plants as they may have powerful medicinal potential. It is very possible that the "weeds" in your garden may be more valuable than what you are trying to grow. Seek out local native healers where you live to help identify native plants.

Farming is a noble profession in which we serve the Lord and our fellow man. Genesis 2:15 says:

> *And the Lord God took the man, and put him into the Garden of Eden to dress it and keep it.*

Please carry on this tradition.

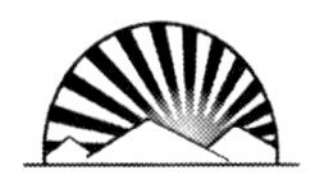

Chapter Eight: **Ideas We Simply Overlook**

There is a great deal more to regaining a state of wellness than by using natural self-administered methods such as enemas, major dietary changes and supplements. However, those three modifications in most any lifestyle will lead to better health. The following considerations are presented after many years of research, personal trial and feedback from others.

The first three influences listed below are a lifetime pursuit and open to much discussion and reflection. There is a current fancy medical term designed to impress called "psycho-neuro-immunology" of which much as been written about. Plainly speaking, it is referring to the brain/body link as well as the spiritual side of healing. It is our mission to attempt to de-mystify all therapies and teach something simple.

I: PERCEPTION

A change in "perception" means a different way of looking at things, such as how we see ourselves, and our purpose—our personal life journey?

You must forget about holding on to negative events of the past and forgive yourself and others for not being perfect.

Over many years of interacting with many people with life-threatening illness, a common thread has appeared. At some point, previous to the acute stage of the illness, an event occurred that was perceived as being so negative that life was no longer joyful. The messages we give ourselves, no matter how subtle, permeate every cell in our bodies, which are holograms of the whole. This event may have been the death of a loved one, a break up in a relationship or marriage, a business failure, or any personal expectation that didn't turn out as hoped.

Illness is a very acceptable way of committing suicide, especially if the illness is cancer or one of the big money diseases. Our minds program our bodies just like a computer—"garbage in - garbage out".

In addition to all physical changes needed to promote natural healing, we need to make mental changes. This could begin by asking and answering the following questions, and we will not get the right answers until we ask the right questions:

1. WHAT IS THE PURPOSE OF MY LIFE?

The mentality of most people with illness is to give power and responsibility to a doctor who will hopefully provide the magic remedy which will eliminate the illness without causing any disruption in lifestyle or thinking and insurance will pay the bill. Why not? Only when we become uncomfortable enough will we ever be open to change—we love our comfort zone. However, most people who are ill are split into more than one person. Most people work at a job that provides them with no self worth except to make enough money in order to live another life away from work. Is the purpose of life to work and consume?

People with illness who can redirect their life into service instead of consumption stand a better illness survival rate.

2. AM I MORE THAN MY BODY?

Current evidence from many cultures seems to indicate that the spirit that resides in our body survives outside the physical body. Some people have experienced "out of body" experiences. Our present in-body experience on this earth, in this place, in this culture, cannot be mere random selection. Why are some born to poverty and some to wealth? Why are some born to white and some to black? Why are some born to deprivation and some to privilege? It is conceivable that our present life situation could be the result of events and actions occurring over generations—the fruit of which is ours to bear. If this is so, then there may have been and still are lessons to be learned during the body experience. It is time to break any negative ties to the past and to secure a better future for generations to come in right action and word in the name of Jesus.

II: PRIORITIES

A shift in our priorities should result after proper introspection, such as, am I willing to partner with God and take control of my personal health or give this power away? Is consuming all that life is about or can I learn to exercise restraint?

If we can shift our "perception" of who we think we are and begin to forget about our ego, then we are open to changing our priorities. There is an old saying that a person on his deathbed never says "I should have spent more time at the office".

Let's get real here...In order to regain and maintain wellness, we have to *change*! Change what? The answer is whatever has produced an imbalance—either self imposed or imposed by others.

Regardless of how dedicated we may become to a life of service, we cannot help anyone unless we help ourselves first. *The buck stops her*e! You must become the best person you can be both physically, spiritually and emotionally before you can help anyone else.

The first "priority" is to ask God for the strength and guidance needed for personal transformation. Become like the pebble falling into the pond and create a ripple effect outward from yourself. *Change*! When you change, others begin to change around you.

III: **COMMITMENTS**

Partnering with God requires that we be obedient to His Word and faithfully accept our responsibilities. In other words, in order to regain/maintain wellness we need to make and keep our commitments.

Presumably, after self-examination through introspection and prayer, there begins to surface the core values of whom we really are. If we dare to strip away the mask of the person we have been pretending to be, if we dare drop this ego and mind set of pretense which has steered our life patterns, then we are ready to allow the person God created us to be to prevail.

A rewarding, healthful, fulfilling life means keeping the commitments of your core values. What are these commitments? We do not dare to presume that the path of one is the path for all. Some commitments might be:

- I will seek the Lord in all things.
- My job is to be the best person I can be.
- I will become more loving and understanding of others.
- I will direct or redirect my life in order to make a positive difference.
- I will change my lifestyle to reflect my core spiritual values.
- I will continuously search for inner truth from the Holy Spirit within.
- Money will no longer be the primary reason for actions.
- I will lighten up and laugh more.
- Words are not actions. I will walk the walk, not talk the talk.
- I will be open and receptive to uprooting strongholds that prevent growth in me and others.

We have only lightly discussed your personal journey. There is much more to be said and learned. Each personal path is different. Realization of our purpose is the goal. Creating a partnership with God to live a life of service is ultimately, in my opinion, the most satisfying and healthiest way to live.

IV: **A Consistent source of pure water and air - environment (**See Chapter 2)

V: **Fresh, chemical free food raised and prepared with love (**See Chapters 2, 4)

VI: **Daily physical exertion** such as rebounding, walking, stretching and daily quiet time in prayer or meditation of at least 1 hour daily. (See Chapter 6)

VII: **Elimination of over-stimulation of your digestive juices.**

Under the "Mayr Method" of coming off an intensive cleanse (Appendix G), I spoke about the importance of chewing. However, there is one big exception to this that includes eating between meals and the practice of chewing gum. Eating between meals may be necessary at times if you are diabetic or exerting lots of energy. Our body, however, prefers to function in a regular rhythm. That is why eating our meals at the same time each day is a healthful practice. By not confusing our digestive system it can be better prepared to do its job when it knows when to do it.

Chewing gum has become another addiction that just causes more harm to the chewer and only benefits those who make it and sell it, along with dentists and doctors. There is nothing redeeming about its ingredients. In fact, its sugar and other contents (intended to stimulate and to give us a jolt) are what keep us coming back for more. What is this oral fixation that civilization has with cigarettes, gum and snacking? I am sure that the answers could fill several more books. But, for our purposes now, I need to emphasize that when we chew unnecessarily we are over stimulating our digestive juices to work when they are not being utilized. This can result in ulcers of the stomach and an eventual a break down and loss of enzyme production when they are actually needed. When we overuse something or over wear something it becomes worn out more quickly. Our digestive system is critical for life and health in our body. We should preserve it and not abuse it as God has intended so that we may live longer and prosper in His service.

VIII: **Replacement of silver/mercury fillings, root canals, and metals in mouth.**

Mercury can cause a huge laundry list of problems in the body too numerous to mention here. Many of these symptoms can easily be misdiagnosed and difficult to treat without giving due consideration to the possibility of mercury poisoning. Mercury migrates from the tooth into your body and brain via several pathways. If you are suffering from a chronic illness it just makes good sense to eliminate this toxic and negative contributor to your overall well-being. Just get rid of it!

Silver/mercury fillings have been around a long time and are still offered as the cheaper alternative to less harmful materials. In the long run, it is not worth endangering your health to save some money. I recommend to all my students that they go to a knowledgeable and understanding dentist who knows how to remove your old fillings safely using what is called a “dam” to prevent swallowing mercury in the process.

A **root canal** is a dental procedure commonly used to remove dead or dying nerve tissue and bacteria from inside a tooth. Something (?) is used to disinfect or kill the nerve and then a sealer is used to fill the area. According to some health conscious dentists, the original bacteria can not be permanently removed and will eventually return and travel to other parts of our body despite whatever toxic substance was suppose to kill it in the first place. All this is done in an effort to save an unhealthy dying tooth at the expense of acquiring some other chronic problem. Is it worth it? It is probably worth it only to the dentist.

The best defense against losing your teeth is a healthy diet, regular brushing and flossing. If a problem arises, Rose can attest to the fact that holding your fresh urine in your mouth for twenty minutes at a time and then spitting it out (since it draws out the toxins) along with a couple of drops of Oreganol (oregano oil) on the infected gum area can resolve an abscess or gum infection and restore the health of your teeth. Do this two or three times a day for two or three days as a first line of defense.

When Rose hesitantly went to a dental clinic to have a tooth pulled, she was seeking some assurance from an unknown dentist by asking several questions of him. Instead of answering her honestly and with concern he acted annoyed with the attitude of "either let me pull it or get out". After ignoring her for some time, he refused to treat her and she was asked to leave and not return. This insensitive and un-Christian like attitude was very upsetting to Rose, at first, until she treated the problem herself and has had no further difficulties since after almost five years now. Truly, God is good! Whether or not we recognize it, He often saves us from ourselves and opens the door to other alternatives.

IX: **Recognizing toxic irritants in the home and workplace**, such as air ducts, carpets, cleaners and waxes, molds and mildew, radon, lighting and harmful energy fields from high voltage power lines and electronic devices like TVs, cell phones, computers, microwave ovens and food prepared with aluminum foil. Even those products used for personal hygiene come under question and especially cosmetics—all of which may be transferring unhealthy substances through our air passages and the pores of our hair, nails, scalp and skin.

What is our obsession with covering up odor with more odors or simply surrounding ourselves with all kinds of scents? Common sense should tell you that it takes a chemistry set and/or laboratory to produce these smells that, in my opinion, are causing adverse effects on our health. More and more people are developing sensitivities to made-made products and few actually recognize that what they are using is the source of their health problem. Haven't you ever felt overwhelmed and uncomfortable being near a person wearing a strong scented cologne or perfume? If we need to cover up our body odor, then perhaps we need to clean up our body internally? Furthermore, have you ever felt ill spending too much time in a newly carpeted or painted room? Headaches are common when over-exposed to toxins released in our environment.

The only exception I take to the subject of an over-scented society is that of Aromatic Therapy and the natural scents found in nature. Certain smells have been found to be very beneficial. The trouble is that the clever people who are marketing products to us are aware of this and have exploited these scents in combination with chemicals. Don't confuse these unnatural imitations with the pure essential oils of the flower used in Aromatic Therapy.

X: **Don't be misled by advertising...**

Reading Labels is essential to knowing if a product is more harmful than good. If you do not know what an ingredient is, look it up before buying. Learn the "red flags" such as *propylene glycol* and *sodium lauryl* (or *laureth*) *sulfate* found in most cosmetic and personal care products such as shampoos and toothpastes.

Many words in advertising are being misused on packaging by stretching the truth. When you see the word "natural" you expect to get the real thing such as real fruit, not just some natural flavors. Many "natural" fruit drinks are merely highly sweetened water with so called "natural flavors" added.

The over consumption of white sugar is one of the major hidden causes of illness. We begin to hear this time and time again. However, it doesn't quite register until you gain some understanding as to why. White sugar turns most easily into alcohol, which is the greatest enemy of calcium in our body's chemical equation. White sugar depletes the body of needed calcium used for the proper digestion of protein. Unutilized, undigested protein when not eliminated is stored in the bloodstream, organs and cells of the body. It has been shown in laboratories that all that is needed in a petri dish to grow cancer cells are sugar and acid—an acidic animal protein. Really *think* about this! In a predominately meat-centered and driven society over-run with sugary breakfast cereals, drinks, desserts and alcoholic beverages, what are the odds of getting cancer, let alone diabetes or one of many other illnesses? Are you willing to gamble with your life and the life of your family?

Sugar comes in many disguises. High-fructose corn syrup is a "biggie" to watch out for as well as all kinds of malts. Remember to read the percentages which may only apply to a portion of the container. Twenty-eight grams of anything is equal to an ounce. So if there are twenty-eight grams of sugar to a double portion container that more often than not is consumed as a single portion, you are really taking in two ounces of sugar. To be really conscious of labels—if we can even trust them—it is best to carry a small magnifier in your purse or wallet. Better yet, if you can not read it, just forget it. What is it that they do not want you to know?

XI: **Avoiding soy products:** For years now, soy has been purported to being the ideal protein substitute for non-meat eaters or as a healthy alternative for anyone. I encourage anyone who doubts what I am about to say to do some research on your own. One place to start is on the website of the Weston A. Price Foundation and "Soy Alert": www.westonaprice.org/Soy-Alert/ (although pro-dairy). Don't just rely on the many untruths of the producers, marketers and lobbyists who gain to benefit from public gullibility. Much research has been done but you will rarely hear about it since corporations have too much to lose. Unfortunately too, third world countries who are asked to grow it are using land that could otherwise better feed their people with more traditional crops instead.

It is often said that the Asian cultures have benefited from a soy diet for hundreds or thousands of years. What they don't tell you is that soy is consumed by Asians in very small amounts as a condiment and not as a meat replacement and that the soy was fermented in a traditional way that neutralized toxins—unlike the modern methods used today. Their particular health benefits came from other sources in their overall diet. Another untruth is that soy is a complete protein. Like all legumes, soy beans are deficient in sulfur-containing amino-acids methionine and cystine while its fragile lysine is being lost in the food processing. A third untruth, worth drawing attention to, is the claim that fermented soy foods are a good source of B12 for vegetarians. However, researchers say that the compound resembling B12 can not be utilized by the body and that consuming soy actually increases the body's need of B12.

So much more can be said about soy food products and soy processing than I intend to say here. Certainly, an entire book can be written if it hasn't already been done. I would like to summarize some of the key problems resulting from an over consumption of soy in the diet and let you investigate further if it concerns you and leave you to draw some conclusions for yourself. Remember, responsibility starts with you and a desire to find the truth. Don't just take my word for it either. The lobbying interests on both sides will present a confusing case.

Soy Alert on the above mentioned website brings these points to light:

- Soy increases the body's requirement for vitamin D
- High levels of phytic acid in soy reduce assimilation of calcium, magnesium, copper, iron and zinc—Soy foods *do not* prevent osteoporosis.
- Trypsin inhibitors in soy interfere with protein digestion and may cause pancreatic disorders.
- Soy phytoestrogens disrupt endocrine function and have the potential to cause infertility and to promote breast cancer in adult women. They also have the potential of causing thyroid cancer and autoimmune thyroid disease in infants. Megadoses found in soy formula are implicated in the increase of premature sexual development in girls and the delayed or retarded sexual development in boys.
- Soy processing today results in the formation of toxic lysinoalinine and highly carcinogenic nitrosamines—like the nitrates found in processed foods I spoke of earlier.
- MSG, a potent neurotoxin, is formed during soy processing and typically more is added to mask the strong "beany" taste of textured vegetable protein

products (TVP). Both soy protein isolate and the TVP produced from it is used extensively in school lunch programs, commercial baked goods, diet beverages and fast food products and form the basis for many food bank programs in Third World countries. Obviously it has proven cost effective for corporations both prior to and after we fall ill.

- Large amounts of herbicides are being used in the U.S. on genetically engineered soy beans. This certainly does not benefit us or the environment.

Seeking soy as a "quick fix" substitute for animal food is not the healthiest solution. What is needed, instead, is a lowering or elimination of protein consumption from *both* animal and soy bean sources.

Still, you may possibly disagree with these findings since there are many pros and cons to be found on the Internet. Just keep in mind that too much of anything, even if it is good for you, is *not* a good thing. Variety in your diet is an excellent way to ensure balance and good health.

XII: **Changing to non-restrictive natural fiber clothing and underclothing.**

Chemicals are also present in man-made fabrics as well as in all new fabrics in which the coloring is set and should be washed prior to body contact. Fire retardation is also made possible with chemicals. Not only do we need to become aware of hidden substances that we may be sensitive to, but we need to allow for all parts of our body to breathe when choosing clothing. Of course, this last comment will hardly appeal to your worldly fashion sense but it may affect some health conditions that are prevalent today....

Candida and fungus such as jock itch and athlete's foot thrive in dark, warm, moist conditions. Wearing loosely fitting, moisture absorbing and quick drying cotton fabrics will minimize the problem. Close fitting underwear and slacks may also contribute to sterility in males. Tight clothing actually serves no purpose other than to draw attention to our sexuality. An overemphasis on sex in our society is bringing us into a downward spiral. It is one thing to want to look clean and pleasing to the eye and it is quite another to become a total distraction and the object of lustful thought and action. If we truly want to reflect our Christian values to the world and have a positive effect on others then we need to dress accordingly.

XIII: **There seems to be evidence that "sun staring" recharges our batteries**. I mention it here as a point of information. I have not studied it thoroughly nor have I had enough experience of my own to recommend it. However, the sun is a vital source of energy for all living plants, animals and humans without which we couldn't survive. I believe that the practice of sun gazing is well worth investigating. One rather complete source of information can be found on this website: http://sungazing.vpinf.com/. Some people may derive health benefits if done regularly while others may not. This is not for everyone. Certainly, if done improperly, it may be harmful as well. Please attempt it only if you feel personally guided to do so, with full knowledge of what you are doing while accepting full responsibility for your actions.

XIV: **The Insurance Factor**

In our present day socio-economic climate, the Insurance Industry creates strong influences on our everyday lives. When realizing the fact that the Insurance, Banking, Chemical/Pharmaceutical, Agro-business and Medical industries are all tied to each other by the money trail, one begins to wonder where personal integrity went.

The most well-meaning, AMA physician, with great personal integrity is a product of a system that is governed by money, greed and power. A license to "practice" a medical art in this country carries with it the stipulations that licensee agrees to "practice" this art according to the accepted standards. The Boards of Medical Licensure only accept one standard and that is whatever is currently taught in the schools funded by the Insurance, Banking, Chemical, Pharmaceutical and Agro-business industries. Should a licensed physician deviate from the norm, the license will be taken away. Should a trained physician endeavor to help sick people without a license, he/she might be arrested for breaking a law by "practicing" medicine without a license. I keep putting the word "practice" in quotes because that is exactly what happens to you as a constant laboratory animal in the industry of organized medicine.

When you purchase any kind of insurance, you are participating in a lottery. You feel that you are going to become "ill/sick" at some time and so you buy medical insurance. The insurance company hopes that it can collect lots of money from you and not have to pay out anything or pay out much less than you paid in, and it sets guidelines as to how much it will pay and for what. So let us say that you become ill/sick. Why did you pay all that money to the insurance company or HMO if you never intended to get something in return? Once you begin to use your insurance you are trapped in a money-driven model of health.

We are all subject to a physical mishap along the path of life in the body. Do we buy auto insurance for maintenance? Most of us buy auto insurance for an accident when the car needs to be put back together or patched. Everyday maintenance of our bodies should be a personal responsibility taught early in life, and insurance should only be purchased for the traumatic accident or major crisis, if at all. Self-insurance is much cheaper.

As I sit at my computer in Belize writing this manuscript, the United States is caught up in a heavy debate about universal health insurance and the extreme costs of providing it for most Americans. Taxes are likely to increase to offset these costs and everyone is anxious as to how the final outcome will affect him or her personally. If Americans were to make healthier diet and lifestyle choices both individually and for their families they would not need constant Rx maintenance. Major illness is on the rise today and it is especially evident in our youth, who are becoming obese, and developing diabetes and other complications at a very young age. This crisis as well as all major illnesses can be prevented if we can have the courage to set ourselves apart from the maddening crowd and create a new norm. Corporations and businesses, large and small, will have to adjust to the new growing demands of a health-conscious society. If we stop buying whatever is thrust upon us as the latest and greatest, mouth-watering and satisfying sugar and/or sodium overload, we would begin to see other options being offered to us. This applies to all aspects of our society and mass merchandising.

Medically speaking, our present day society seems to say “life in this body at all costs”. The Medical/Industrial Complex keeps devising drugs and procedures to prolong life in the body. Are we creating a generation of weak people kept alive by drugs, implants and artificial means? Are we honoring God or just playing at being a god?

When we can reject medical insurance and put that money into better food, lifestyle, and self-improvement, when we can reject dependency on anyone for health-maintenance, then we have taken a major step toward personal empowerment and enlightenment.

XV: **Your Personal Remedy for Health…**

The ancient therapy discussed in the following section is an essential tool for all students of natural healing to learn and employ. When combined with the other skills taught in this Guide it will produce results that will amaze even the most skeptical.

Urine is not, as commonly believed, the excess water from food and liquids that goes through our intestinal tract and is ejected from the body as "waste". What it actually ***is*** may surprise you…

When you eat, the food you consume is first broken down in the mouth, then in the stomach and eventually in the intestines into extremely small particles called molecules. These molecules are then absorbed by tiny tubes in the intestinal wall and pass through into the blood stream. The blood circulating throughout your body then becomes a vehicle for these food molecules and other nutrients. Along with vital immune defense and regulating elements such as red and white blood cells, the blood carries antibodies, plasma, microscopic proteins, hormones, enzymes and more—which are all produced and transferred from different locations found throughout the body.

As our blood circulates, it passes through the liver where toxins are removed and later excreted from the body in the form of solid waste. Let me repeat something incase you just missed it—toxins are removed and later excreted from the body in the form of solid waste. Meanwhile, our blood, which now has been purified by the liver, continues on its journey to the kidneys. When blood enters the kidneys it is filtered through an immensely complex and intricate system of very tiny tubes called nephrons. When passing through these tubes the blood is filtered or shall we say "squeezed" under great pressure. This filtering process removes excess amounts of water, salts and other elements in the blood that your body does not need, at the time, and are then collected within the kidney in the form of a purified, sterile, watery solution called urine.

It should interest you to know that many of the components of this "clean" watery solution called "urine" are then reabsorbed by those same tiny tubes within the kidney and delivered back into the bloodstream. Think about it! Would God have created this normal functioning of our organs if it were not beneficial to our body? So, what we now have left over, that our body has no immediate need of, is passed out of the kidneys into the bladder where it is excreted.

The kidneys have the precise function to keep the various elements in your blood balanced. When your body doesn't need something at a particular time, it is excreted—not because it is toxic or bad for the body, but simply because the body is not in need of that particular element at the time. Urine is composed of 95% water, 2.5% of urea and the remaining 2.5% is a mixture of minerals, salt, hormones and enzymes.

A Powerhouse for Profit…

It is common knowledge among medical researchers that many of the elements of the blood that are found in urine have enormous medicinal value. When these elements are reintroduced to the body they boost the body's immunity and stimulate healing like nothing else does. Research is going on all the time in laboratories throughout the world where technicians are looking to isolate certain components of urine in order to create new drugs and profit from them and they do—by the billions. Don't be misled by the name of a drug or the ingredients you read on a label. If you were to seriously seek answers as to where these were derived from (and nobody ever bothers) you would discover that these pharmaceutical and cosmetic laboratories are creating their own concoctions from what already exists in nature so that they can put a patent on it. You can not put a patent on urine. Urea (2.5% of urine) is packaged in expensive creams and lotions because it has been medically proven to be the world's best moisturizer. I suppose that most people prefer spending lots of money and lavishing themselves with creams rather than the idea of giving themselves a urine massage. This is because we have been manipulated to have a certain mindset, not only in regard to our own urine, but one that convinces us that we need to have these products to be beautiful and healthy. These products are too numerous to mention and I am refraining from naming names but I would bet that each of you reading this book would find something in your own bathroom cabinet that fits this description.

Dr. A. H. Free, one of the founders of Miles Laboratories, published his book *Urinalysis in Clinical Laboratory Practice* in 1975 where he refers to urine as being sterile and containing thousands of beneficial compounds of which here is a partial list:

> Alanine, Arginine, Ascorbic acid, Allantoin, Amino acids, Bicarbonate, Biotin, Calcium, Creatinine, Cystine, DHEA, Dopamine, Epinephrine, Folic acid, Glucose, Glutamic acid, Glycine, Inositol, Iodine, Iron, Lysine, Magnesium, Manganese, Melatonin, Methionine, Nitrogen, Ornithane, Pantothenic acid, Phenylalaline, Phosphorus, Potassium,

Proteins, Riboflavin, Tryptophan, Tyrosine, Urea, Vitamin B6, Vitamin B12, Zinc/

Some of these names may be difficult to pronounce while others may still be recognizable to you. Think about this statement: Each of us is manufacturing and carrying around our own natural and personalized medicine.

Desperate measures in desperate situations?

Not only is urine entirely sterile after secretion but it has an antiseptic effect as well. I can remember Rose telling me that she was watching a segment of the TV show, "Survival", when one of the reality show tribe members was stung by a large jelly fish. He immediately asked another tribe member to urinate on the effected area. Somebody had their wits about them! Perhaps this incident on television helped to raise people's consciousness as to the natural survival techniques we all have the ability to utilize. We needn't be stranded on an island to benefit. I have personally used urine on cuts and bites and stitches after surgery to speed up the healing process and to prevent infection.

During our lifetime, each of us has either heard of or read of a "life or death" story where one or more individuals were trapped in places without food or water for days at a time. Those that survived expressed the fact that they had drunk their own urine. Those that did not drink their urine died. The deceased probably could not overcome their misconceived notions that their urine was a waste product of the body. They did not understand that urine is a substance of beneficial elements that is secreted when the body is overloaded with them. Remember that the kidneys job is to keep our blood in a healthy state of balance by eliminating too much of a good thing.

I would certainly suggest that if you were one of those people caught up in a life or death situation by all means drink your own urine or even someone else's for that matter. However, under normal circumstances, it is most advisable for you to do so only if you are a reasonably healthy individual eating a healthy diet and you do not use chemical drugs or allopathic medicines. This is because you would be reintroducing more of these toxic substances (that the body has already eliminated) back into your system—once again, throwing the body out of balance.

Urine therapy is a method based upon the principle of 'natural cycles'. As long as we do not interfere chemically with the body's natural cycle, the body produces urine which is perfectly suitable for re-cycling. If you ingest a great deal of chemical substances then they will end up changing the composition of your urine. These substances can come from processed foods as well as your medicine cabinets or local drug dealer. Normally, urine is a healthy substance which contains healthy, harmless and nourishing components—not harmful chemicals. I believe in the value of urine therapy but do not usually recommend it until after a student has cleansed their body well enough and changed their diet.

Urine Therapy is to be taken seriously. It has brought relief to people suffering with multiple sclerosis, colitis, lupus, rheumatoid arthritis, cancer, hepatitis, hyperactivity, pancreatic insufficiency, psoriasis, eczema, diabetes, herpes, mononucleosis, adrenal failure, allergies and so many other ailments. There have been numerous books and reports written and studies done that confirm its health benefits. One needs only to look on the web to learn more about it. It has been practiced since ancient times. The only reason that you do not hear more about it today is because there is no money to be made from its use and billions of dollars would be sacrificed if everyone were to utilize their own natural medicine.

Keep it in mind, also, that urine contains elements that are very specific to the individual from whom it comes such as antibodies, enzymes, hormones, and other natural chemicals specifically made by the body to regulate functions, correct imbalances and combat diseases. It is anti-bacterial, anti-fungal, anti-viral, anti-neoplastic (anti-cancer), anti-convulsive, and anti-spasmodic. The idea of consuming your own urine does take some getting used to—which is mostly a mind game. Once you overcome your own resistance and try it, you will discover (if your diet is clean) that it actually can be quite pleasant and certainly tastes better than other medicinal remedies. In fact, if you are consuming large quantities of water it may not have any taste at all. Rose and I encourage you to consider using your own urine as outlined below, both internally and externally. We never recommend anything to others that we do not already employ ourselves in our regime of natural healing.

Please refer to Appendix H: How to apply Urine Therapy.

XVI: **Bathing in a Rainbow of Healing Energy...**

A healthy body requires a source of "healing energy". Let me relate to you how I became interested in this subject:
The year was 1980. I was training as a chef's assistant under Brother Ron Pikarski, a Franciscan monk. He was hired the same time as me by an award-winning natural food restaurant in North Miami Beach, Fla. Brother Ron had recently won the Cooking Olympics in Belgium. He won with a vegan creation, an Olympic first. I was also teaching natural healing part time which interested another chef friend. He told me of a scientist he knew who was

working in the field of "Bio-Magnetics". This was beyond my comprehension then and so my friend brought me some very simple literature describing how certain vibrational energies are compatible with the human body's natural frequencies and some vibrational energies are not compatible. I read the literature and soon met the scientist, who personally taught me the science behind his work. I was so impressed with the undeniable principles of truth behind Dr. Louis Barbara's work that I became a close friend and devotee until I moved out of the U.S. Unfortunately, at this time, he is aging and may even have passed on at the time of this writing. His research in energy healing has not been fully appreciated in his lifetime.

Dr. Barbara taught me: Everything in our cosmos, everything in our solar system, everything in or on the planet earth has a frequency, which he called "resonance". A frequency can be a number that indicates how many cycles per second (hertz) any object is vibrating. And, believe it or not, everything is vibrating. A rock, for instance, has a frequency but the molecules that comprise a rock are usually moving imperceptibly slow.

Dr. Louis Barbara was hired as an electrical engineer by Bell Laboratories in the 1940s to work in vacuum tube research. He is reputed to have discovered the phenomenon of "white noise". He learned to measure frequencies and built (in a home lab) several rudimentary instruments that he used to treat various ailments of friends by using electrical energy or frequency as a healing energy—thus validating the theory of an "energy healing."

An illustration of how it works…

An excellent example of vibrational resonance is the tuning fork and the piano tuner. The tuning fork has a built in frequency or vibration of resonance when struck. The piano tuner keeps adjusting the tension of each string so that the note struck is in harmonic resonance with the specific tuning fork. Eventually, when the string is "tuned" and the note is struck, the tuning fork will vibrate on its own through resonance. When the piano is in tune, it is putting out sound at its full potential.

Our bodies get out of tune...

When our bodies are "out of tune", we are like storage batteries—a unit of rechargeable electric cells—that are wearing out. Like a storage battery, our body has a built in charger. The human body is 80% water with electrolytes that need constant charging to keep all components working harmoniously. When we get fatigued outwardly, our inner workings also become fatigued similar to what happens when an electric motor tries to run on low voltage. Eventually, the motor will burn out.

Our "body battery" functions best when it is able to receive the natural energy from the molten magnetic core of our planet Earth and the cosmic energy from the sun and Solar System and beyond. We also are recharged by constant chemical reactions in our body resulting from breathing clean air and eating vital foods—all part of an energy healing process.

Dr. Barbara determined that the natural harmonic frequencies of a healthy human body correspond to frequencies found in nature including visual, auditory, olfactory and tactile. These healing frequencies, according to Dr. Barbara, are the frequencies of the visible light spectrum, or the seven visible colors in a rainbow. In today's modern world, we are being constantly exposed to man-made frequencies, resonance and vibrations that are not compatible with a healthy body, such as microwaves, artificial light, electrical appliances and power lines. In addition, we tend to insulate ourselves from natural healthy energy by using concrete, rubber soled shoes, carpeting and man-made fiber clothing. Eating energy-dead food and the negativity of our thoughts also contribute to a body electric that is "out of tune".

Harvesting energy frequencies for healing...

When two wires—each conducting some kind of electrical energy—are placed parallel to each other, the space between the wires contains a magnetic or energy field. Dr. Barbara realized that the brain produces delta, theta, alpha and beta waves of energy, but alpha energy ranging from 8–10 cycles per second (hertz) is the optimum frequency for the healing change. Using the alpha energy as a baseline and adding the frequencies or cycles per second (hertz) of the colors of the visible light spectrum, primarily red, orange, yellow, green, blue, lavender and violet, Dr. Barbara began building devices which would use these frequencies in parallel to produce a "pulsating magnetic field." Furthermore, he was able to isolate negative, positive and biphasic or neutral magnetic fields for specific energy healing uses.

Why color vibration?

Dr. Barbara concluded that the vibratory rates of the colors of the visible light spectrum are compatible to our body's organ, gland and electrical systems. When the body is subjected to these frequencies over the alpha baseline, the body is gently guided into a matching vibration by resonance much like the tuning fork vibrating when the note of the same pitch is struck on the piano, sort of like "bathing in a rainbow". When I was a small child I always heard it said that there was "a pot of gold at the end of a rainbow". Have you ever heard of anyone finding that "pot of gold"? If you could somehow manage to be in the right place at the right time and be immersed in the refraction of sunlight hitting the ground at the end of the rainbow, I believe you would be instantly healed of any illness—if reaching that spot were achievable.

Now, the above information may be confusing at first read. It took me many readings of Dr. Barbara's theories to finally grasp what he was talking about and this was only the beginning. Finally, after many visits from Arkansas where I was living beginning in 1983, I agreed to have Dr. Barbara build for me the first "Soma-Mag" Energy Regeneration System based upon a prototype I experienced in his lab. This energy healing equipment is available only at our retreat in Belize to experience by our students interested in this energy healing research.

To my knowledge, this first piece of equipment is a one of a kind, as no others were built like it. There is so much information on this subject to relate that it will have to be added in several sections, over some time, perhaps on our website. Please check there for further updates. There is also much written by others in the areas of color and light therapy. For the serious researcher, we would like more collaboration in these areas of research. To inquire or contribute further regarding energy healing, please contact us via our website: www.naturalcleansingtechniques.com

XVI: **Native Medicinal Plants and Healers**

Here in Belize we are fortunate to have a wide diversity of medicinal plants but they are rapidly vanishing due to destruction of their natural habitat and the death of most of the old native healers. Fortunately, one old Mayan healer left a legacy here. Drs. Rosita Arvigo and Greg Shropshire came to Belize in the 1980s and through their efforts and apprenticeship with this same Mayan healer, have preserved most of his knowledge by way of books and practice.

Our present day world has already lost thousands of species of indigenous plants that could help reverse illness. On every continent, in every country there are a few rapidly disappearing native healers with knowledge of local plants that have been used to heal for generations. Very few are preserving this knowledge or propagating these plants for future generations. Native healers die off without passing on their priceless knowledge. Seek more information about medicinal plants where you live and those who employ them.

In our opinion, using the natural plant material that God has created is far superior to the extracted concoctions that laboratories synthesize. They fail to understand that the natural essence of the plant is only effective in combination with other vital ingredients found in the plant as a whole. Pure is better than with added impurities. Fresh is better than unnaturally preserved. However, if you can not grow or harvest your own then dried herbs and tinctures are available from reliable companies such as Frontier Herbs, Rainforest Remedies or North American Herb and Spice.

My wife and I are far from experts in this area but we are gradually learning and applying what we learn to our health maintenance. As we landscape and cultivate our garden beds, we look to discover the beneficial plants that spring up unbeknown to us and preserve them. An informative reference guide for recognizing medicinal plants where we live has been *Rainforest Remedies* by Rosita Arvigo and Michael Balick. Around our home we have acquired Jackass Bitters, Cowfoot, Red Head,

Oregano, Papaya, Wild Sage, Wire Wis, Vervain, Periwinkle, Amaranth and more with no effort of our own. Others, such as Avocado, Coconut, Aloe Vera and Soursop we planted ourselves. Even if you do not have the convenience of nearby plant life, it is wise to become familiar with what can be found in areas that you intend to visit—especially if you are a hiker, camper or an explorer of the great outdoors. You never know when it might come in handy. Survival skills are an art to be cultivated and possessing similar books relative to your neck of the woods or places of interest would be well worth having.

Putting ideas into practice...

Remember, that regaining ones health is like detective work. You should thoroughly explore one idea at a time. If you try to do too much at once then you will never know what worked and what didn't. That is why we advise starting with a basic program and then gradually introduce new ideas, one at a time, for further improvement while keeping in mind that it may take several weeks or months to discern a result from natural methods. Patience and persistence is the key and not flitting from one idea to another.

Lifestyle changes take time. As you learn new skills and develop healthier habits of living it will become second nature. If you are feeling overwhelmed, step back and slow down but don't give up. It is far better to progress slowly and steadily than to carry a heavy load, rush and collapse along the way.

One must have continued faith and deep commitment to overcome a serious illness. Negative thinking or complaining to others will only backfire on you. No one likes to hear a friend or loved one say how much discomfort he or she is in without trying to do something about it. As a result, you may find yourself being pressured to take a different direction than the one that you have chosen. Only confide in those who are totally supportive and can encourage you during any difficult times. Oftentimes, when the body is being restored at the cellular level and the cause of your problem is being eliminated, your symptoms are the last to disappear. You will experience a mini healing crisis in the process as we have discussed before. This is the time to stay positive and be thankful to the Lord.

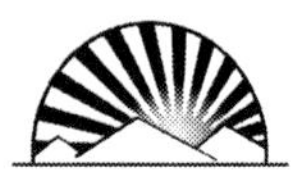

Chapter Nine: **Bringing It All Together…**

Initially, I challenged you, the reader, to set your self apart by taking a stand for what you believe and putting it into practice. By healthful eating and lifestyle changes, you set an example to others and begin to initiate changes in our society. Individually, by first changing ourselves we can change others in our immediate surroundings like the ripple effect of a pebble in a pond. When like-minded people come together, the power in numbers is multiplied and we have a greater impact on how things are done. Rather than just allowing all that is being done to us to continue, we need to influence the way things ought to be done—producing healthier lives, a healthier planet and actively participating in the preparation for God's Kingdom on Earth.

This chapter is devoted to the stimulation of ideas that we hope will provoke discussion and then some action from the simplest step, such as stopping buying certain products, to the more challenging steps such as speaking out to your congressmen and corporate and local business owners and/or re-evaluating your priorities and starting anew—with Jesus Christ alongside anything is possible.

Some thoughts may seem repetitive but well worth emphasizing…

The Question for Today Is Still, WHY?

I can remember my earliest attempts at using the word, "why" in question form. As a very small boy, the realization was soon grasped that adults never appreciated being asked "why" and especially not more than once, which in my generation usually ended with a "because I said so" declaration of parental authority.

If the question "why?" is asked often enough, even to currently accepted answers, we can usually begin to get at the "truth". During my adolescence my gut feelings were that most adults did not want to explain the essence or truth of many situations because it threatened their comfort zones somehow. When you ask "why?" often enough of government or industry sometimes you may uncover a money trail with questionable morality, as in recent corporate scandals.

Each of us has many questions not yet answered lying dormant. I encourage you to begin each New Year with at least one "why?" For instance, my first "why" for 2003 came from the lead article in an issue of *Rural Arkansas* distributed by my rural electric-cooperative. At that time, it seemed that our "Electric Co-ops and University of AR Medical Sciences (UAMS) had teamed up to promote and support The Community Cancer Control Program to reduce cancer incidence and mortality in rural areas of Arkansas." The Rural Electric Co-ops were providing the grant and use of their offices to conduct cancer-screening procedures. UAMS trains healthcare professionals who treat eighty-percent of the state's population.

Why? The answer then and now is the same—because the business of testing for cancer is not only profitable but also leads to more profitable treatments. Why don't we focus on reducing cancer incidence rather than testing and treating symptoms? Why don't we reduce medical costs dramatically by teaching people how to detoxify their bodies and then nurture them to heal naturally?

Do not buy into the cancer industry's pleas for more research money. In 2002 I wrote the following article for a local newspaper:

The Race for the Cure

The public consciousness is once again being stimulated in order to reap financial support for Cancer research and its protocols for which the past seventy years have produced high profits but no cures.

Cancer was being cured in the 1920s and '30s and is being cured today by simple natural methods. But, the medical cancer industry prevented then and now dissemination of the knowledge and promotes its own profitable industry of research, surgery, radiation, testing, chemotherapy and drugs all of which treat symptoms not causes.

Cancer has steadily increased because we continue to poison our air, water, soil, food and thus ourselves. Our bodies are designed to overcome disease, but when they become overwhelmed with toxins, our resistance fails.

The Insurance industry dictates which profitable protocol is acceptable and since most people have bought into the insurance lottery because they do not want to accept responsibility or change their lifestyle if they become sick, they give that responsibility to an industry driven by profit not cures.

Having healed myself of colon/pancreatic cancer in 1969/70 and having taught hundreds of others natural methods, I know that by changing lifestyles and diet, by learning ancient and modern self-administered techniques, most anyone with desire and commitment can heal naturally of Cancer and other degenerative disease. If too many people did this, it would be bad for the economy.

Cancer is not a disease, just one symptom of a society out of balance. Excluding trauma, we cause our own illnesses and have the God-created ability to heal naturally if we are willing to assume personal responsibility for every aspect of our lives. Cancer has its roots in agriculture, industry, ecology and personal integrity. The billions of dollars being raised for research by "racing for the cure" is a prime example of the cancer of greed within the Healthcare Industry. There must be a new paradigm which I believe is a return to the principles of moral integrity exemplified by the Christian family farm upon which America was founded.

And a Question of WHEN?

When are people going to wake up to the fact that we are constantly being manipulated by the media, who are being manipulated by the money-hungry drug companies, research laboratories and the AMA and countless lobbyists who want you to believe that cancer is a disease that requires some scientific cure requiring huge fundraising—money that certainly could be put to far better use for humanity. Unfortunately, nowadays, the Golden Rule has come to mean, as Dr. T. Colin Campbell put it in *The China Study*, "he who has the gold makes the rules"—rules that guarantee more profit.

The truth is that cancer is the body's own defense mechanism for dealing with a body out of balance—plain and simple. Recovery is achieved with personal lifestyle changes; detoxification and rebuilding of healthy body tissue. Once again, this requires an individual to make a commitment and to act responsibly. The trouble is people do not take the time to nurture their bodies at the expense of giving up some pleasure or convenience. They actually take far better care of their automobiles.

There isn't now, nor will there ever be, a quick fix to our health problems, either with drugs or by going under the knife. These can only be temporary fixes unless, of course, what caused the imbalance in the first place has also been eliminated. I suspect that most cancer survivors have somewhere along the way made lifestyle changes as well. The ingesting of drugs alone increases the toxicity of the body and depletes the natural immunity to fight off illness.

The real disease exists in a society that refuses to change and submits to the overpowering influences all around us. People overindulge in work, in play, in food and in drink. Their bodies are over toxic, over stressed, over weight and spiritually deprived.

We all have the seeds of cancer. This is not an overnight occurrence that you may catch as if it were a cold. Different bodies respond in different ways to a gradual (most often since childhood) build up of imbalances in their body causing an array of so called "diseases" including cancer.

What we really need isn't universal health care but rather universal health education on a physical, mental, emotional and spiritual level—creating a society that is more ethically and morally balanced and not driven by the love of money but rather by the love of one another. Jesus said, in Matthew 22:37–40:

Thou shalt love the Lord thy God with all thy heart, and with all thy soul, and with all thy mind. This is the first and greatest commandment. And the second is unto it, Thou shalt love thy neighbor as thyself. On these two commandments hang all the law and the prophets.

Regardless of your own religious beliefs—should you be reading this book for the health benefits alone—what righteous person can argue against love and all the good that is derived from it?

Going "green" not only saves our planet but it restores our health. Finding alternatives to unhealthy practices, household/business and consumable products in our everyday lives will accomplish so much more now and for generations to come than the "race for the cure", which I believe only lines the pockets of some and can actually save the lives of few.

By supporting these fundraisings we are also encouraging the status quo…an unhealthy mindset that perpetuates illness and a diseased society—will we ever wake up to change?

Defusing untruths...

I am constantly finding articles in the news that shock and baffle me. One such item recently in the news was about a 27-year-old woman who was about to have both breasts removed as a preventive measure to cancer since her gynecologist told her that she had a breast cancer gene that apparently ran in her family with a history of such cancer. What appalls me after reading this article is the fact that so many in our society are frightened by the word "cancer" as a result of scare tactics used by the medical establishment.

Cancer is merely a symptom of a body out of balance and it is not something you can simply cut away. We all genetically have the predisposition to some kind of illness. If we are fortunate to know beforehand where our weakness lies than we can take preventive measures – even without knowing of any weaknesses we should do the same. The body is designed to work perfectly under the proper conditions, thanks to our Creator, unless those conditions are drastically altered. With today's lifestyles being what they are, we are continually trying to push our bodies to perform and expect to stay healthy despite numerous unhealthy conditions—such as unclean air, water, food, improper diet, stress from work and dysfunctional relationships. These and more, as previously discussed, contribute to a body out of balance producing symptoms of illness.

I immediately left my personal comment to this article as follows:

> Dear Lisa, you have been brainwashed by the medical establishment. Just because you have a gene you need not get cancer or any other symptom of illness if you are willing to change your diet and lifestyle now. By learning to cleanse and detoxify your body and switch to a plant-based diet, you can prevent and cure most all illness. Don't be trapped by your insurance into making a decision you will regret forever and do not allow fear tactics to overcome common sense and trust in God.

People today are obsessed with their bodies but mostly for the wrong reasons. There exists this fascination in the news with the latest and greatest diet fad. Gimmicky diets, emphasizing one particular food or another, are another form of misleading information that can possibly cause more harm in the long run. With short term practice, you may lose those extra few pounds but at what cost?

Eventually, you will put them back on while possibly further exacerbating your body in being out of balance. By depending on some new form of diet food such as a cookie to fill you up while eating less is not helping to establish good eating habits for long term health. Once again, people marketing these products and gimmicks are counting on you, the consumer, to seek a quick fix solution that satisfies your unhealthy cravings. I can not stop you from throwing away your money nor can I force you to make healthy choices. My mission is to hopefully influence you to think and act responsibly when it comes to taking care of the temple of God—your body. Applying common sense to lose weight and to stay fit doesn't cost you a small fortune.

Drinking ourselves to death...

Oh, you say, “but I do not drink”. I am not just talking about alcohol. It goes without saying that the over-consumption of alcohol is a killer. Furthermore, I have already discussed the problems with contaminated sources of our drinking water. What I am seriously concerned about here, that bears special emphasis, relates to our consumer habits of consumption and the untruths in advertising.

By allowing ourselves to be victimized by clever and deceiving marketing we are killing ourselves and our children. Until now, I haven’t as much as hinted about the devil, but Satan is cleverly infiltrating our mind, body and spirit on a daily basis simply by thrusting unhealthy, devalued, high calorie, fat, salt and sugar and sugar and more sugar-filled bottled and canned drinks at us—even concentrates on the shelves, in the frozen food department or worse yet, at the fast food counter. We all get thirsty and we are telling you of the need to drink at least half our weight in ounces of liquid (ideally pure water) each day. So, it is tempting, not to try this “made from natural...”

drink or “fortified with...” product without ever looking at its list of ingredients and their percentages?

The problem is that the Devil knows exactly how to fool us into making wrong choices. He is the great deceiver who has been around since the Garden of Eden. The producers of these products think that they have something new and improved to offer but just to be sure that you like it and that you will come back for more they add tempting flavors and very addictive sweeteners and who knows what else? As we unsuspectingly and quickly gulp down these beverages we become hooked; throw off our body chemistry; interfere with food digestion; gain lots of weight; develop diabetes and other physical ailments including cancer; upset our emotional balance and our ability to receive spiritually because our minds are befuddled. Are we to invite in the Holy Spirit and to expect Him to take up residence in a chemically altered and unclean temple?

If you do nothing else but eliminate these undesirable drinks from your diet and drink plenty of pure water between meals, you will be on your way to better health.

Rebuilding you and society from the ground up...

Much of this book has already dealt with illness and wellness and we surely pray that you have been stimulated by the ideas presented giving you the capability of achieving health stability. Without your personal health, you cannot live out your potential and God’s plan for you. So, take charge of your health, please.

Back in Chapter Six regarding stress, I told you about the infamous Dr. E. who felt that in order to be “successful” you first had to establish financial stability.

That advice would be good today if you were mostly money driven. I would suggest today that you just need to "establish stability", period.

First, we must feel secure in the love and protection given freely by God to those who know Him. Next, we need to develop our personal repertoire of skills to become as self-sufficient in every way possible. Third, we need to seek out like-minded people to join or form community. And finally, we need to become grounded in a church and fellowship and worship together. Does this sound "old fashioned"?

Perhaps we should consider returning to those days of yesteryear when the pace of life was slower and more meaningful, even before TV. Could it be possible that civilized mankind came to a fork in the road of life's choices and went down the wrong road?

This morning, as I relish my morning breakfast of yesterdays—vegetables with pasta—leftovers, I am contemplating how the Industrial Revolution which brought about massive distribution of soda pop and breakfast cereals, has robbed people of their health in western style societies—now propagated all over the world. In fact, most all processed food, most every product produced in a laboratory and even in our favorite restaurants are either devoid of real nourishment that our bodies can use, contain toxins and over-dose us with sugar, sodium and calories we don't need.

Of course, it is not just the food but an over-paced and stressful lifestyle that puts modern day convenience of "fast" food and ease of mobility way ahead of healthful food preparation at home along with daily exercise.

We have become pawns in this game of life where we are subject to mass media and advertising that continually entices and tempts us to believe their untruths. News headlines, for instance, are sensationalized and easily misinterpreted to suck you in, but how many of us actually read the whole story? Our shortened attention span prevents us from taking the time to investigate the catch phrases plastered everywhere, especially on food and other product packaging. Is it their fault or our fault or both for making us ill?

Responsibility needs to be spread all around in a society where we actually exist solely to survive and/or to amuse ourselves with pleasure or puff ourselves up with pride via our accomplishments. This may sound adequate for some, even desirable for others. I have been there and I have done that, but I have now come to discover that life can be richer and more meaningful and beneficial to others when we include God. America has gradually stripped God from its very foundation—no longer in our Pledge of Allegiance, taught in our schools or exercised in our government. I urge non-believers who struggle with and experience a void in their life to look to Jesus Christ for their answers. And to all my fellow Christians, we can do more by first changing ourselves and setting an example for others, thus becoming a force to reverse trends in our society. Industry can be and is a good thing when utilized wisely and in everyone's best interest and not just for the greedy few at the top.

If we could retrace back to sometime in the 1800s we could perhaps find the beginning of the Age of Industrialization. That is the fork in the road of which I speak. I believe that the "industrial giants" of the 1800s took us down the wrong fork in the road. We need to retrace our steps, heal and rebuild the earth behind us that we have messed up and return to the path of a more earth-friendly lifestyle.

Visualize, if you will, a world run by energy obtained from more earth-friendly sources like wind, waves and tides, the sun and the earth (solar and geothermal). Picture a world not run on oil. Picture a world without internal combustion engines that spew out toxic fumes. Picture a world that is in harmony with nature rather than one which is trampled on by the will of man for profit. And finally, picture a world that walks the talk of the greatest commandments—"Love the Lord thy God...and love thy neighbor as thyself." (Mat 22:37-39)—that is my vision for a better tomorrow.

Can we achieve my vision? Yes we can. I suggest to you that the way to achieve this vision is to re-shape our society, not by a Mao type revolution but by a spiritual and cultural revolution. The foundation and backbone of America was and still remains the Christian family farm. America was originally a one-of-a-kind experiment. It was founded on biblical principles and the teachings of Christ. These principles were the foundation of the family, the community, the Constitution and the government. Very little of our original foundations are evident today.

Our Christian morality has been diluted and polluted by consumerism. Our families have split up due to financial pressures. Our family farms have been ousted by multinational, corporate agro-business. Return again to another important fork in the road that greatly influenced future society. I am speaking this time of the industrial effort expended to supply our military in times of war. Mothers were called from their role in the home to produce in factories for the war effort, giving rise to a whole generation of children raised by nursery schools and baby sitters. Home schooling gave way to government approved education which separated church and state.

I believe that this is the time to begin a whole new direction...

How and Why to Set Your Self Apart...

I have always been curious and somewhat fascinated by people who choose to be different. We now live in a private Mennonite community. The Mennonites and the Amish came from the same roots. They have chosen to live apart for generations. It is not my intention to propose the Mennonite life for everyone, but they set a good example for us to follow in many ways that I would like to relate to you. Life is far from perfect in a Mennonite community or any community. However there is a basic blueprint or model here for us all to learn from. First, let me give you some interesting history about where we now live.

Spanish Lookout is Belize's most modern Mennonite town settlement located in the north-western part of the country. Mennonites run their own church-based communities as a self-sufficient people while practicing strict traditions. In keeping with these old cultural ways of life, they live in a reserved manner maintaining the use of their Dutch/German dialect and their homes and clothing reflect their simple and conservative tastes.

Who are the Mennonites?

Mennonites are a branch of the Christian church, with roots in the radical wing of the sixteenth-century Protestant Reformation. Part of the group known as Anabaptists (because they re-baptized adult believers), the Mennonites took their name from Menno Simons, a Dutch priest who converted to the Anabaptist faith and helped lead it to prominence in Holland by the mid-sixteenth century. Modern-day Mennonites number almost one million worldwide, with churches in North and South America, Africa, Europe and Asia. Mennonites are known for their emphasis on issues such as peace, justice, simplicity, community, service, and mutual aid.

In keeping with their spiritual roots, Mennonites still believe in a close adherence of the Scriptures and a personal spiritual responsibility as the basis of their faith. Radical from the beginning, but later considered conservative in many of their beliefs, Mennonites have come to represent a spectrum of backgrounds and ideologies.

Pacifism is one of the cornerstones of the Mennonite faith, prompting many young Mennonites to elect service to the church rather than military service. The Mennonite church emphasizes service to others as an important way of expressing one's faith. A disproportionately large number of Mennonites spend part of their lives working as missionaries or volunteers helping those in need, both nationally and internationally, through agencies such as the Mennonite Mission Network or the Mennonite Central Committee.

Mennonite migration began in Europe; then to all provinces of Canada; then Chihuahua, Mexico; Belize; and South America—everywhere linked through marriage. Each of the elders of the different families still living, all, I am sure, have wonderful stories to tell of their particular journey toward freedom of religion and choice of lifestyle still being practiced and enjoyed today. When first arriving in Belize—then British Honduras in 1958—they did not ask for land grants or tax exemptions but agreed to pay all duties and taxes. They asked for and received the freedom to educate their children in their own schools, exemption from military service as well as from compulsory social programs. They promised to pay all expenses of establishing their own community and to take care of their old and infirm—they would not become wards of the state. Imagine that! No wonder my wife, Rose, and I have been invited to become involved in their community.

Life in Spanish Lookout...

Celebrating its fiftieth year in March of 2008, Spanish Lookout has, for the most part, been integrated into the Belizean way of life, and this community coexists with other ethnic groups. They are the major producers of dairy, poultry, vegetables and beef, and supply the entire country with these commodities. Quality Chicken—Belize's most popular chicken—is located in Spanish Lookout as well as a new-comer called Fiesta Chicken. Gradually we are beginning to see more naturally raised beef, lamb and chicken become available for health-conscious consumers too. Western Dairy, Belize's only commercial production of milk is also located here. Furniture manufacturing and house construction are two other important economic activities of Spanish Lookout, and people will visit in search of tires, car parts or machinery, as the prices are some of the most competitive in the country.

Located in the Cayo District of Belize, this Mennonite settlement is spread over open fields and rolling hills, with large trees that have been around for centuries. Over the years, since first settling in this area, several thousand acres of bush and jungle had to be cleared by the Mennonites in order to make the land more productive. Now, small houses with zinc roofs, as well as some modern ones dot a countryside that resembles a scene from a rural town in the

Midwestern United States or perhaps in Pennsylvania. Cornfields and cattle pastures can be seen for miles. Part of the main road is paved, but most are good gravel roads. The main road is lined with gas stations; tire supply stores, farm centers and mills. People from all around the area come to the Farmer's Trading Center, informally referred to as FTC, for groceries, household goods and supplies. Having its roots as the local general store, this community-owned-and-operated business has been thriving and expanding.

Men and women are all busy at work whether in the home, on the farm or at their place of business. Children, when not being schooled or just taking time out for play, are always helping with the house and farm chores. Young boys are trained early to drive tractors. The entire community seems to focus on "production" and the care of the family. It is a common occurrence to find folks here coming to the aid of another family, church or community member when in need. The women have regular get-togethers to help one another sew quilts or to make blankets and clothes for the needy. They are hard working people yet always friendly and willing to help.

Today, residents of Spanish Lookout realize the growing importance of cultural understanding and unification amongst the people of Belize and others worldwide. Thus, they do welcome tourists who are respectful of their lifestyle and are mindful of how they themselves dress and act when visiting.

Transformation in Belize...

God has blessed us with the opportunity to learn from and to exchange ideas with the Mennonites. Rose and I are developing emotionally and spiritually from our experiences and growing fellowship with our sisters and brothers in Christ.

Rose, having an open mind and always a seeker of truth was led to her Lord Jesus in this community and was baptized in the Belize River on March 30, 2008. Raised as a Reform Jew and having an Orthodox grandfather who was president of a large temple in New York City, she too was guided by the Ten Commandments and mostly Jewish family tradition and didn't experience a personal connection with God except perhaps as a "big brother". However, her closest friends in school were not Jewish and this always kept the question of Jesus in the back of her mind. As adults, we were both led in our search (as too many of us are) to investigate a so called "holy" man in India. Leaving no stone unturned, we traveled there and actually discovered most of the teachings of Jesus.

Rose had a prophetic dream while staying at the Ashram in 1992 that has remained clear in her mind until this day. At last, fifteen years later it all began to make sense—she was being shown her eventual spiritual path. In her vision, she saw three men walking toward her that she had recognized as being Moses, this particular "holy" man and Jesus—one teaching had led to another, until finally coming to rest in the love of Jesus, here in Belize. It began while familiarizing herself with the Old Testament and the history of the Jews, Rose spent many hours in friendly exchanges of fellowship with a Christian brother in Spanish Lookout—questioning and listening and re-questioning. After much of her reading, it had become quite apparent that Rose was highly disturbed by the knowledge of the behavior of the Jews during bible times and of the Pharisees own self-righteousness. Later when told by a visiting pastor from Mexico that God had a plan to use Rose to heal people, she felt unworthy and immediately was impelled to read the entire New Testament for the first time and then research the web for the pros and cons of accepting Jesus as the Jewish Messiah. The strongest objection that she found was the claim that Jesus did not bring world peace. In John 14:27, Jesus states:

> *Peace I leave with you, my peace I give unto you: not as the world giveth, give I unto you. Let not your heart be troubled, neither let it be afraid*

Rose felt that the opposing Jews were looking in the wrong place and expecting world peace at the wrong time—it is yet to come when Jesus returns. Many of the other claims seemed to her to derive from an ever-present stubborn refusal to see from another perspective. It became very clear to Rose that she wanted to be baptized and declare Jesus as her Lord and Savior. The veil had been lifted completely for her and now we continue this journey together in His service.

Each day here is a new beginning, learning to be more like Him with each other and with those whom we come into contact with. Life for us would be shallow and self-indulging if we didn't hold on to this goal.

Naturally, what is most fulfilling about living here in Spanish Lookout is the fact that we live in a God-centered community. Much of life revolves around the church. For some there is a strict adherence to certain practices according to inherited translations of the Bible. For others there has been a breaking away from a more rigid church life of yesteryear in order to seek a non-legalistic but an abiding and more personal relationship with Jesus and Father God. Earlier I said that there are no perfect communities. Here too, we find a struggle to contend with old and new ideas among its many churches and even within families whose members have stopped going to the same church. Although set apart, we still find a microcosm of difference that abounds in the world today. However, there also coexists a strong desire to heal the emotional wounds and to inspire spiritual mending, after all, most everyone in Spanish Lookout is related one way or another. This may take some time, perhaps another generation, but we are optimistic that eventually this community can bring it all together for everyone's sake and the establishment of God's Kingdom on Earth. We must all learn to live together and love one another and not sit in judgment—only God can do that.

I am especially fond of the close family that is well represented here. Families typically average six to ten children. Our closest neighbor raised fifteen beautiful children. A family farm takes help and cooperation from everyone. All hands young and old are required to carry their fair share of the daily workload. Babies are often nursed or carried on the hip while mothers work goes on indoors or outside. Meal preparation and cleanup along with laundry are ongoing daily activities requiring all females to participate. Nursing and nurturing of the young are carried on long past most other "more civilized" cultures. The focus of most families is first on God, then on each other within the family and then reaching out to serve others.

Our church sponsors a Saturday sunrise men's breakfast and study circle twice a month. The agenda is to watch a video, followed by discussion, and breakfast together. Last year we watched several videos by an elderly pastor well known in the U.S. teaching the responsibility of the man as the head of the household and the nurturer of the women under his care. I was particularly moved one Saturday morning by the message this pastor taught on the sacredness of virginity. Growing up as a teenager in the U.S. was quite different than here. The lesson taught me about virginity by my parents was, "Better not get her pregnant". How different is the message in a God-driven society! The virginity of the female and the male are respected and nurtured until the union and bonding are as one within the sanctity of marriage by the spilling of the blood of the female on the male during first sexual penetration. This precious blood union and the teachings of the family and church leading up to a marriage—I believe, as God intended—is the spiritual and physical foundation upon which to build a family, a society and a country.

Rose enjoys and benefits from attending a bi-monthly meeting held by the women of our church that includes women of other churches as well. Their first priority is always to uplift one another in spirit and come together in prayer for those in need. Then they break up into smaller groups and review and discuss either a chapter of a book or some other written material they have all been reading that challenges them to be better Christian women, wives and mothers. Afterward, they share in some snacks and good fellowship.

Besides multiple church events and gatherings within the community, at least once a year there are family gatherings with grown children and their children, grandparents, aunts, uncles, and cousins enjoying good times, traditional Mennonite food and fellowship. Visiting relatives and being visited creates a steady interchange between Canada, Mexico, Belize, Bolivia, Brazil and elsewhere.

Although this is an agricultural community, there has been little emphasis on the growing and eating of vegetables. As a result, their body chemistry is out of balance and there has been much illness and death, even in the short time that we have lived here. Rose and I are trying to raise their consciousness, as well as yours, to the importance of a healthy diet. Although there are no fast food restaurants and fancy coffee shops, junk food has a way of creeping in. Sugary soda pops and "juices", candies and packaged junk food are everywhere in Belize. There is an over dependence on animal food such as chicken, eggs, meat and dairy since it is what they produce for the rest of the country. Until the farmers are willing and able to find alternative ways to earn a living and provide healthier food choices, the health of the Mennonites and Belizeans will continue to suffer.

Another problem that we hope to overcome here is the use of pesticides and herbicides that are poisoning the land, the animals, the food, and water supply—all contributing to chronic illnesses. According to Charlotte Gerson and Morton Walker in *The Gerson Therapy*, "The fundamental damage starts with the use of artificial fertilizer for vegetables and fruit as well as for fodder. Thus, the chemically transformed vegetarian and meat nourishment, increasing through generations, transforms the organs and functions of the human body in the wrong direction."

I have offered my knowledge and experience of organic farming to anyone interested, free of charge and I will continue to do so. I am only one person hoping to make a difference in a small community. You and the countless others who may read this book and everyone that you come in contact with, all together, have the increased power to affect change within your own communities and in nations if you just make up your own minds to very selectively use your buying power to do so. Industry will have to eventually adjust to the consumer's demands.

Releasing old habits takes self-control...

While Rose and I partner with God in our efforts to transform others, we continue to be transformed ourselves by the love of God and the examples being shown to us in this community. Change is never easy and I do not believe that one can do it alone. First, you have to desire to change and second, you need to ask Jesus or Father God to help you. Habits are hard to break and strongholds of the mind are deep rooted. In order to uproot them, you must immediately plant new seeds and allow them to take root, eventually overtaking the old.

Remember the old adage, "practice makes perfect". However, we are all sinners and we know also that "to err is human". We must acknowledge our mistakes, ask for forgiveness and begin anew.

Don't think of your new food choices as a life-long diet of deprivation but rather as a life-giving alternative to eating yourself to death.

Be willing to step out of the box you have been living in and be willing to rethink everything...question and re-question your own tightly held ideas as well as those of others until you discover real truth for yourself.

Setting Yourself Apart from the Seeds of Cancer is not meant to imply that you go off and live in a cave somewhere. What we are talking about here is...

- Partnering with God

- Having the desire, courage and determination to raise your consciousness to a Godly level and live by your convictions

- Practice self-control of worldly desires

- Effect change in others by first changing yourself

- Personally taking the necessary steps to increase your health physically, mentally, emotionally and spiritually with better lifestyle choices

- Bringing meaning and purpose into your life through service to others as a way of serving God

- Helping to establish His Kingdom on earth as living examples of Christ's teaching. This will draw others to Him.

I could go on and on, but I feel these summarize the main ideas which reflect that you ought to not just go along with the crowd and what is popular—be your own person and the best person that you can be. In this way we can all help to eliminate the seeds of cancer in ourselves and in the world today.

Good health is more than just diet. It is a delicate balance of which "attitude" plays a big part. This crazy world could be such an amazing place if we would all put this into practice and learn to accept our differences without casting judgment and blame. If you choose to do things differently, don't let others discourage you from what they do not yet understand. Set an example instead and be a leader. God uses leaders to show others the way.

Paul listed nine godly virtues that constitute the fruit of God's spirit—the inward and outward effect of the Holy Spirit taking up residence in our body—His temple. Galatians 5:22–23:

But the fruit of the Spirit is love, joy, peace, longsuffering, gentleness, goodness, faith, meekness, temperance: against such there is no law.

The word "temperance" refers to restraint or self-control. Certainly, it takes a lot of self-control to practice and achieve the other eight virtues—all of which contribute to good health of the body and of the planet and the entire world population. When all those who have chosen to set themselves apart are united as one, this world will be a far better place than it is today. Together and with God's help we can make it happen. We can begin to create God's Kingdom on earth while paving the way to an eternity in the Kingdom of Heaven.

The Bible says, "Because strait is the gate, and narrow is the way, which leadeth unto life and few there be that find it (Matt. 7:14). Are you willing to be among the few or are you going to be among the masses to whom God will profess, "I never knew you: depart from me, ye that work iniquity" (Matt. 7:23)?

Our prayer for each and every one of you is that you will continue on a path of physical, mental, emotional and spiritual wellness—one that includes Our Lord, Our God as your personal teacher, guide and partner; practicing the discernment of truth from worldly untruth and discovering your own unique gifts that will give purpose to your own life and joy to both yourself and others.

Start today by *Setting Yourself Apart*.

Rose and I would like to close this book with part of a forgotten prayer we learned from Wendell Berry in his essay "God and Country" from his book *What Are People*

For? Here, Mr. Berry quotes from the prayer "For Every Man in His Work" in the 1928 *Book of Common Prayer*:

> *Deliver us, we beseech thee, in our several callings, from the service of mammon, that we may do the work which thou givest us to do, in truth, in beauty, and in righteousness, with singleness of heart as thy servants, and to the benefit of our fellow men.*

In Jesus name we pray, Amen.

Appendix A: **Instructions for Taking an Enema**

It is most desirable to take the coffee enema early in the morning and it may be repeated again in the early afternoon and/or evening, depending upon the toxic condition of the body. Enemas using coffee late in the evening may interfere with a sound sleep, and if needed at that time, many people prefer to use only warm purified water for their enema, omitting the coffee.

The materials needed are as follows:

- Organic, regular, non-instant, non-decaffeinated coffee (see sawilsons.com)
- Coffee percolator or ceramic/glass/stainless steel/enamelware pot (NOT aluminum or teflon)
- Purified water
- 2-quart enema bag (or see Appendix B for making your own canister)
- 30" colon tube (28, 30, or 32 Fr diameter)
- enema tip for colon tube (optional)
- ice cubes from purified water (optional)
- sheet of plastic to line floor where you will lay
- towels and pillows to lay on, and/or exercise mat
- organic extra virgin olive oil for lubrication (in a small pop-top container for convenience)
- toilet paper
- liquid castile soap (for colon tube and bag clean up)
- hanger and clothespin (for hang-drying colon tube)

The best procedure is to arise each morning earlier than normal to allow time to take the enema in a relaxed, unhurried state. The steps for proper procedure are:

1. **Preparing the coffee** (30-40 minutes**):** We have learned after talking with Scott Wilson who specializes in making a unique light-roasted organic coffee blended just for enemas, that regular perking in an automatic electric

percolator cycle is not long enough to extract enough essentials. It was recommended that the coffee and water be placed in a stainless steel pot, brought to a boil, simmered for fifteen minutes, cooled and then strained. If an electric percolator is used, allow it to cool and re-perk a second cycle or use a stove-top coffee pot and perk slowly fifteen minutes. Drip coffee makers are unacceptable. Always use coffee at body temperature.

My wife and I prepare our two pots of enema coffee the evening before. This way, each of us only has to warm the coffee to body temperature for use in the morning. When doing an intensive cleanse, prepare another pot of coffee after your a.m. enema so it will cool down for use later in the day or evening. We leave it in the pot, covered on the stove until needed since we have been advised that the coffee is okay if used within twelve hours of brewing.

Coffee must be brewed in enamelware, corning ware, glass, or stainless steel. **Do not use aluminum or Teflon** at any time! Use 3 rounded tablespoons of coffee grounds to 2 quarts of purified water. Anytime water enters into the body, it should be non-chlorinated and filtered or purified. Those who have a tendency to become "jittery" or nervous from coffee should use a weaker solution of only 2 tablespoons of coffee grounds per 2 quarts of purified water. A 12-cup stainless steel, stove-top percolator is the most convenient pot to use. Once the coffee starts to perk, turn down the heat and allow it to perk for 15 minutes. When planning to make another pot full right away, we draw more benefit from the first portion of coffee grains by only needing to add 2 tbs. to the already perked grains and then proceed to perk it an additional 5 minutes (20 min. total). If you do not own a percolator, you can use any stainless steel pot with a lid that will hold 2 quarts liquid—Place water and coffee in the pot, bring to boil, simmer 15 minutes, strain and cool to body temperature.

2. **Preparing your colon:** Should you have the luxury of preparing the coffee fresh and then waiting for it to cool down, it is desirable to do some form of mild exercise such as stretching, rebounding or brisk walking. This exercise is more likely to result in a normal bowel movement prior to your enema. The enema is much more effective if the colon has been evacuated.

A helpful option is to first take an enema with warm purified water. This begins the cleansing of the colon, removing large particles of residue and most of the gas. When this is completed, you are ready for the coffee retention enema. The warm water enema is optional and does not need to be taken if you can retain the coffee enema for the desired length of time. You'll need to discover what works best for you.

3. **Preparing your equipment** (5 minutes)**:** This is not a sterile procedure, in the medical sense, but it needs to be very clean.

Designate a stainless steel saucepan of 2 quarts or larger for your personal enema use. The enema tip on the end of the hose attached to your bag or canister is not adequate to give a "high enema". You will require a colon tube 30″ long and 28, 30 or 32 Fr (diameter). Place the colon tube in the saucepan, cover with 2–3 inches of water and heat until the water feels very hot with first indication of minute bubbles at the bottom but definitely not quite boiling. We want to preserve the rubber and make the tube last as long as possible—it is costly to obtain. The rubber, when continually over-heated, will soften, stretch and expand and become more difficult to insert.

To help sanitize equipment, pour off this hot water through your enema bag or canister into the sink while retaining the tube in the bottom of the pot. Close the clamp or cut-off valve and add 1–2 quarts of the special blend coffee. Double check the temperature—if it is still a little overheated, you can cool it down with purified water ice cubes. When satisfied, open the valve again to release just a little bit along with any trapped air bubbles. With your enema bag in one hand and your colon tube in the now empty pot in the other, you are ready for the next step.

4. **Getting into position:** Prepare a pallet on the floor of the bathroom near your commode using a large enough piece of plastic covered with old towels and 1 or 2 pillows for your head. It is also advisable to use an exercise mat on the bottom for extra comfort. I generally prepare my mat first so that it is waiting for me upon my arrival with the coffee.

Hang your enema bag near your mat alongside where your hips and knees will be so it will be near enough to reach comfortably for insertion and where you can easily watch the flow of liquid. It should not be higher than 36-inches off of the floor. If it is placed too high, the coffee runs into the colon too fast and under too much pressure, causing discomfort. Sometimes you can adjust the height from a door hook or shower rod by hanging it from the corner of a strong plastic or wire hanger. Most towel rods are at a good height.

Place the saucepan with the colon tube on the floor in front of you while seated on the mat and insert the enema tip into the tube. The saucepan becomes a clean place for removing and replacing the tube after your enema.

Use a little olive oil to lubricate tube and anus. It is non-abrasive and will not damage the rubber. Keep a small amount of olive oil in a convenient pop-top container with a small opening always handy in the bathroom. In final preparation, you may want to make 2–3 wads of toilet paper to use as needed to absorb any leakage. At a critical moment, you can apply pressure against the wad and avoid having an accident during a brief spasm or urge to release. Now you have everything at hand and you are ready to go into position.

The body position can vary to suit the person. The method we employ that is used by most people is to lie on your left side until the solution is out of the enema bag. I was taught to keep my left leg straight and bring my right knee up towards my chest. Rose, on the other hand, prefers to have both knees bent. Try whatever position is most comfortable for you. Slow deep breathing helps to relax you and your internal muscles. You should never try to take the enema while standing or while sitting on the toilet. It is important to remain on your right side with your knees pulled up, for up to fifteen minutes if possible—longer is not necessary. This enables the coffee to reach and stimulate the hepatic valve to open and to release toxins into your colon from your liver.

5. **Performing an enema** (30-45 minutes)**:** Okay, so now you are lying on your left side with at least your right knee bent and you have a pillow supporting your head and neck. Your tube and anus has been lubricated. Hold the end of the tube in your right hand and have the clamp or shut off valve in your left hand. Have a wad of toilet paper handy to place against anus if leakage occurs…

Insert tube in anus about 3 inches and begin releasing the liquid. Continue working the tube slowly into the rectum 24–29 inches. This can be done in a rotating motion back and forth to prevent the tube from "kinking up" inside of the colon. However, do not over-twist in any one direction and always check that your connections are secure before and during this process to prevent an accident with the equipment. Stop the flow if you feel a cramp or spasm to release. When it passes continue this process until the tube is comfortably inserted as far as possible thus releasing the liquid as high into the colon as possible. The tube will move more easily inside you while the liquid is flowing.

If too much of the coffee is released before most of the tube has been inserted you will possibly feel the urge to evacuate. If you didn't evacuate before your enema, you may now need to do so. Rather than struggle at this time, even if only a small amount of coffee was taken in, it is better to remove the tube, relieve yourself and then re-lubricate and try again. This next time, you should be able to work the tube all the way in and successfully get the coffee to reach your ascending colon.

Keep in mind that everyone's anatomy is different, even one person changes from day to day. No two enemas are exactly alike. Some days you may have gas that gets trapped and causes some discomfort and a greater urge to release. Other days you will experience that the tube will kink inside—it hit a snag while going around a bend—which is all very normal. The trick here is to back the tube out just a little bit at a time, slowly, until you see and/or feel the liquid flowing again. Then, in order to go past that same snag, firmly push the tube back in a bit more distance than you had just removed. Of course this only works if you only needed to pull it out 2–3 inches. Just do not give up. You will sense the feel of it and learnt to know what works for your own anatomy. Whatever, you do, NEVER force the tube painfully. This is a painless procedure. If you hit a sore spot, try breathing more deeply and shifting your body slightly. If you still can not insert the tube any further, don't worry about it. Just continue releasing the liquid as much as you can comfortably hold.

After all liquid is released, clamp the tube and remove it slowly with your right hand. Do not pull from the enema bag or canister tubing since this may cause your colon tube to disconnect. As soon as you can reach the top of the colon tube with your left hand, grab it there. For sanitary purposes use a small piece of toilet paper folded and wrapped around the upper tube then slide it down as the tube is removed and catch at the tip to avoid extra handling and leakage from the end of the tube. Then, place the tube in the saucepan.

Roll onto your right side with knees tucked to your chest. Try to hold up to 15 minutes, releasing when necessary.

Remember, each time that you take an enema, it will feel different. Some days you may only hold it another minute or two, while other days you will hold it several minutes or longer. Just do the best that you can. Rose tells me that she may successfully get past her first urge (or spasm) or even a second urge and when she feels that final spasm when it is time to release, she waits for it to pass and then immediately goes to the commode. So, the message here is that you should not attempt to get up from the floor between urges—otherwise you may not make it safely to the commode.

Now, you've come to the best part—just relax and release. Do not rush Mother Nature. The liquid will not be released all at once, even if you think it has. You may feel several spasms over time as it works its way out. Allow yourself at least 15–20 minutes or longer—this makes for more good prayer time and Bible study.

After evacuation, wash out the tube and bag with warm, soapy water, rinse and hang over the tub to drain and dry until next use. This also removes any oily residue that would break down the colon tube's rubber.

You are now ready for your regular daily routine—clean and refreshed! My wife and I start each day this way. When doing an intensive cleanse, we recommend an enema at least twice a day.

Appendix B: **How to Make an Enema Canister**

This is the best alternative to a Fountain Syringe Bag that we know of—created by one of our students here in Belize.

Materials Needed:

- (1) 2-quart translucent plastic pitcher with handle and lid.
- 3 feet clear plastic tubing, ¼″ inner diameter
- (1) Brass hose barb and male adapter ¼ x ⅛ for air or gas hose or match available tubing—¼″ tapered end is best but be adaptable to what is available.
- (1) Clamp or inline shut-off for tubing
- 1 or 2 stainless steel flat washers to match brass hose fitting (½″)
- Brass or stainless steel nut for brass fitting (optional)

Directions:

1. On the outside surface of the pitcher, make a mark directly opposite the handle, just above the bottom.
2. Drill a pilot hole on the mark. Use a drill bit slightly smaller than the threaded end of the brass fitting to enlarger the pilot hole.
3. Slip a flat washer onto the threaded end, heat over flame by holding with pliers, then push into the hole from the outside until the washer firmly contacts surface. The plastic should soften from the heat to permit penetration and seal around the fitting when cooled.
4. A washer and nut may now be applied over the threaded end of the fitting on the inside if needed.
5. Warm one end of the clear tubing in hot water and force it over the tapered end of the brass fitting.
6. Install a clamp or shut-off device on the tubing or just kink the hose to stop the flow.

7. The free end of the tubing can be inserted into your colon tube or an enema fitting can be attached first.

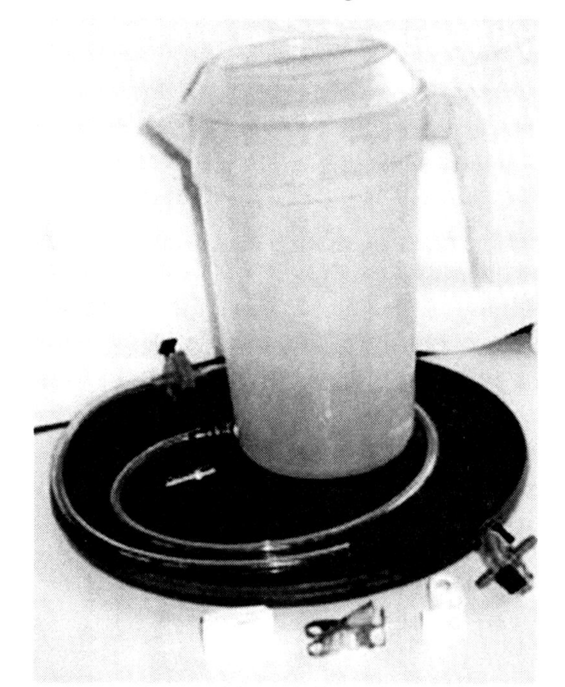

Plastic canister, clear tubing, inline shut-off, misc. clamps

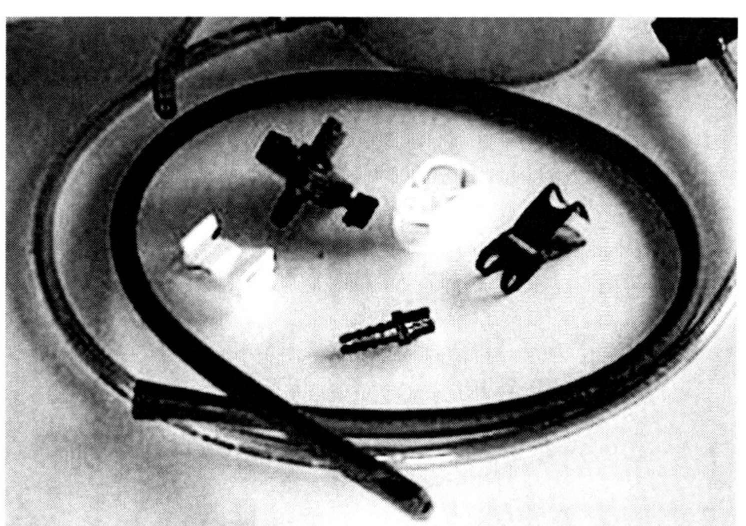

30″ Colon Tube, Brass fitting, inline shut-off, misc. clamps

Appendix C: **Basic Supplements and Supplies**

There are a few items one needs to accumulate ***before*** your Seven-Day Cleanse. Items with an asterisk are recommended to have on hand but are not necessary for the actual cleanse and are spoken of in the section on supplements (pages 88-90).

1. **Minerals**: Min-Col (Daily Manufacturing) or Nature's Sunshine Colloidal Mineral

2. **Rutin** (essential for maintaining healthy blood vessels): Puritan's Pride or Solgar (500mg tablets)

3. **WhiteWillow** (a natural aspirin): Nature's Way (400mg capsule)

4. **Capsicum** (cayenne): Nature's Way

5. **Beneficial Bacteria**: Yeast Away (peakhealthcareproducts.com)

6. ***Oregano Oil**: Oreganol from North American Herb and Spice

7. ***Tea Tree Oil:** Now Manufacturing

8. **Pancreatin**: Now Manufacturing

9. **Kelp**: Algazim by Daily Manufacturing or Nature's Sunshine

10. **Green Food Supplement**: Ultimate GreenZone by Nature's Sunshine

11. **Bentonite Clay:** from Pascalite

12. **Ground Psyllium Seed**

13. **Organic Flax Seed**

14. **Extra Virgin Cold Pressed Olive Oil**—stored in a can or a dark glass bottle

15. *__Epsom Salts__

16. **Organic Special Blend (extra light roast) Coffee** Go to: www.sawilsons.com

17. **Parasite Cleanse**: Para-Cleanse from Nature's Sunshine

18. *__pH Test Paper__

19. **Natural Skin Brush** or loofa

20. **Juicer**: We prefer Green Star twin gear which does not destroy enzymes and vitamins with heat

21. **Enema Bag**: Two-quart fountain syringe douche style or (preferably) a canister (see appendix A)

22. **Colon Tube** (catheter): 30" length x 28Fr. (diameter)

23. **Magnesium Oxide Powder**, NOW brand

24. **Water Purifier**—"Big Berkey" highly recommended but optional

25. **One Pint Size Jar**, preferably glass, with a tight fitting lid for shaking your drink mixture.

26. **One or Two Quart Size Jars** for refrigerating extra juice to be used the same day. You will consume at least 1½ quarts of fresh juice per day.

27. **Food Grade Diatomaceous Earth** (DE) is an optional daily supplement for good health

Appendix D:
Recommended Fruits & Vegetables for Juicing During Seven-Day Intensive Cleanse

Buy ***organic*** whenever possible so as to avoid adding toxins to the body. The following amounts are for ***one person*** for ***seven days*** approximately.

- **20 lbs. carrots**—use approximately 11-12 oz. per juicing
- **5 bunches of celery**— use approximately 2-3 stalks
- **7 tart, green apples**—use ¼ of an apple per juicing
- **3 heads of cabbage**—use approximately $^1/_7$ head per juicing (3 juicings per day)
- **4 or more beets** (depends on size)—use approximately 1/6 beet per juicing
- **3 bunches of parsley**—use approximately. $^1/_7$ bunch (when juicing 3 times per day)
- **4 onions**—use approximately $^1/_6$ to ¼ onion per juicing
- **1 or 2 whole garlic heads**—use 1 or 2 cloves per juicing
- **7 lemons**—Use ½ lemon with warm water each morning for proper pH.
- **7 cucumbers—**Use more depending on other greens.
- **fresh kale** or any green if available.
- **green pepper** if available

At all times, keep your produce well wrapped to avoid loss of moisture and at a cool temperature. ***Freshness is important.***

Depending on the season and the amount of water contained in the vegetables, you will find that the above formula may produce enough juice so that you can save some in the refrigerator in a large sealed jar with each of your first four daily juicings, so that you have enough saved for your last daily cleansing drink and supplements. Obviously, if this is not the case, you will have to juice some more—either juice more each time or juice more often. Make adjustments to the above shopping list as needed depending upon where you live, what growing season it is, and what is available—perhaps the main consideration should be to ideally keep your juices about 50% green (for the live enzymes and alkalinity) and 50% carrot (for the vitamin A/D component that helps cleanse the liver). Beets, preferably fresh, are also important to cleanse and heal the liver.

Appendix E: **Seven-Day Intensive Cleanse**

Before beginning, refer back to pp. 78-81 for more details.
Gather items listed in Appendices C and D.
Start with a Basic Cleansing Diet for several days, then...

Eat nothing other than that which is specified *on the following schedule. If you experience hunger, drink mild green tea or diluted fresh juice. Plenty of liquid is essential.*

Optimum Time Schedule: Repeat for 7 days

6:30 a.m.: Drink 2 tablespoons fresh lemon or lime juice in one cup of water and take 4 Pancreatin caps.

7:00 a.m.: Mix and Drink ***Cleansing Drink***: Place in jar 2 oz. fresh vegetable juice, 8 oz. water, 1 tsp. clay powder, 1 slightly rounded tablespoon psyllium. Shake vigorously and drink before mixture thickens. Follow immediately but drink slowly 10 oz. of ½ vegetable juice and ½ water.

7:30 a.m.: Take **coffee enema**

8:30 a.m.: Take Supplements with diluted vegetable juice: 4 Green Food or 1 scoop green powder, 1 Min-Col, 1 Algazim, 1 Capsicum plus, and 1 *Willow* (Willow is taken just once-a-day) plus ***flaxseed drink** as follows:

> *Soak one tablespoon flaxseed in ¼ cup very hot water, with a secure lid to seal in heat, for eight hours, strain and drink liquid and viscous only. You'll need to press seeds with back of spoon and scrape viscous from the bottom of strainer into your drink. Prepare seeds the night before for the morning drink, and prepare again in the morning for the afternoon drink.

10:00 a.m.: ***Repeat Cleansing Drink***

11:00 a.m.: Take 4 Pancreatin caps with lime juice/water

11:30 a.m.: Take Supplements with diluted vegetable juice: 4 Green Food or 1 scoop green powder, 1 Min-Col, 1 Algazim, 1 Capsicum

1:00 p.m.: ***Repeat Cleansing Drink***

2:30 p.m.: Take Supplements with diluted vegetable juice: 4 Now Green or 1 scoop green powder, 1 Min-Col, 1 Algazim, 1 Capsicum cap.

4:00 p.m.: *Repeat* ***Cleansing Drink***

5:00 p.m.: Take 4 Pancreatin caps with lime juice/water

5:30 p.m.: Take Supplements with diluted vegetable juice: 4 Green Food or 1 scoop green powder, 1 Min-Col, 1 Algazim, 1 Capsicum cap plus **flaxseed drink** (same as at 8:30 a.m.).

7:00 p.m.: ***Repeat Cleansing Drink***

7:30 p.m.: Take **coffee enema** (or earlier is preferred)

8:00 p.m.: Swallow 1 tablespoon extra virgin olive followed by 2 tablespoons fresh lemon juice in one cup of water. Take 4 Pancreatin and go to bed early.

Keep a copy of this schedule close by at all times.

After you have followed this Cleansing Schedule for seven days, choose one of three diet plans in Appendix G to gradually return to regular food. This will allow your digestive system to ease into the process of breaking down solid food—otherwise, you will suffer from indigestion.

Appendix: F:
Considerations for a Seven-Day Intensive Cleanse

The "Optimum Time Schedule" is just that—what you should strive to attain. If you remain focused and get into a rhythm, you will have no difficulty. The problem arises when we allow little distractions to set in and throw us off schedule. It is perfectly alright to start your day earlier. In fact, taking your morning pancreatin enzymes followed by your coffee enema would be more desirable. However, only do this if you can still get your vegetable juicing done in time for your 7:00 AM cleansing drink—earlier is fine but don't push it much later. Remember, early to bed and early to rise is our goal and this is a full days program.

Fit your second enema in where you feel it works best for you—perhaps right after your 4:00 PM drink, at which time, you should plan to have your pancreatin w/water handy if you might still be occupied at 5:00 PM or you might prefer instead, after your 5:30 PM supplements.

Whatever you do, do not become stressed over the schedule. Making minor adjustments is allowed provided you follow certain guidelines. You can make up for a loss of time by pushing your supplement and cleansing drinks a little closer together but do not lessen the time before and after taking your pancreatin which needs to be taken on an empty stomach. Also, bear in mind, that you want the live enzymes and nutrients in your juice to be as fresh as possible. Giving yourself enough time to sort, wash, cut and juice your vegetables (30–45 min) before each cleansing drink is the ideal way to do this program but perhaps not the most practical. When Rose and I do this cleanse together, we share in the prep, juicing and cleanup and save enough juice from each of four fresh juicings in a lidded-quart jar in the refrigerator so we do not have to repeat this procedure a fifth time. Rose is so used to making enough juice for two that when she does this cleanse by herself she only has to juice half as many times.

Depending upon the state of your health, your particular circumstances and available support, you will need to work these decisions out on your own but only make just enough juice for the same day and start fresh the next morning. Not only do you need your juice to be "living" but you need to avoid any contamination from bacteria by keeping your work area as clean as possible. If you can not clean your juicer immediately, then at least remove all the pulp and soak your parts in soapy water until you can get back to it. Wipe your machine and countertops thoroughly of juice and pulp —any remnants left behind will breed unwanted bacteria especially if left on the screen which needs careful brushing. Why expose yourself to more when your aim is to eliminate bacteria and toxins?

During this cleansing process you will lose some beneficial bacteria but we do not replace it until after the intensive program because it would be a wasted effort. The pancreatin, necessary for the break down of undigested proteins, also interferes with a probiotic. We will actively replace good bacteria between cleanses.

Added Suggestion…

We recommend 1 or 2 rounded tablespoons of ***Food Grade Diatomaceous Earth*** (DE), otherwise known as fossil shell flour, every day mixed with water or juice as a supplement to any health program—not as a stand alone "quick fix".
Take this whenever it is convenient for you each day.
Check out: www.earthworkshealth.com for the numerous health benefits and other uses.

Appendix G: **Concluding the Seven-Day Intensive Cleanse**

In order to reintroduce the alimentary/digestive tract to more solid foods after ***each*** Seven–Day Cleanse, a careful regimen must be considered. Either of three different plans may be followed along with the maintenance program outlined below:

Plan I—Hearty Vegetable Soup: Prepare early and eat small amounts throughout the day as desired and chew well. Cook a large variety of vegetables plus potato in liquid with seasoning. When soft, blend ½–¾ and add back as thickener and enjoy!

Continue this for 2 days and gradually add other foods on the Basic Cleansing Diet (p. 81)

Plan II—Mini Diet:

First Day:

Breakfast**:** shredded steamed carrots.
Lunch**:** Large fresh salad with olive oil, lemon/lime juice
Dinner Large fresh salad, one steamed veggie.

Second Day:

Breakfast: Fresh fruit, cooked rolled oats
Lunch: Large fresh salad, one steamed veggie, beans
Dinner: Large fresh salad, one steamed veggie or fresh fruit

Third Day: Start Basic Maintenance Program (p. 271).

Plan III—Modified "Mayr" Intestinal Program: Those with cancer should not use this plan, due to the unmistakable link between dairy and cancer. The modified Mayr program has been used for decades in the world famous spas of Europe for healing and rejuvenation. The principle is that by proper chewing of a specific stale hard roll or type of bread prepared in the ancient manner and accompanied by high acidophilus/lactobacillus milk (diluted yogurt), that mouth and bowel integrity are rejuvenated. This process exercises your chewing muscles; stimulates the flow of saliva and the production of digestive enzymes while reintroducing good bacteria found in diluted yogurt. Specific ingredients are required and a strict protocol must be followed for success.

To prepare for this 3–7-day program, you will need the following: (Do not substitute other products):

1. One loaf of Serenity Farm French Bread (24 oz., round loaf) per day for a minimum of 3 days, but more is better. This may be ordered direct from the bakery by phone 870-443-2211 (Arkansas, U.S.A.)

> **Or:** Bread baked in a wood fired oven (preferable)
>
> **Or:** Hearty whole-grain bread with no bakers yeast, fats, oils or sweeteners.

2. Have available one pint per day per person of (chemical free) **organic plain yogurt.**

Preparation: The bread must be the proper consistency. Remove from bag and cut loaf into eight pieces. Spread these pieces out on a cutting board or cotton cloth to air dry until sturdily elastic in the center but noticeably harder than fresh (1-3 days). Thin the yogurt to a milk consistency with purified water before eating.

Eating method: Just before you plan to eat, cut the bread pieces in thin slices. Pour thinned yogurt into a cup with teaspoon handy. Put a small piece of bread in your mouth and chew slowly until saliva is produced. This retrains your salivary glands. The bread and saliva will begin to form a watery paste with a slight sweet taste. Now, and not before, sip a small spoonful of milk through pursed lips with a slight sucking sound. Mix the bread, diluted yogurt and saliva in your mouth by more chewing and by using your tongue, only now may you swallow. Repeat this process until hunger is satisfied. Any amount may be eaten, however usually 2–3 pieces are sufficient. Take the yogurt by the teaspoonful with the bread mixture in the mouth or not at all. Plenty of water or mild green tea should be taken between meals.

After easing your digestive tract back onto solid food you are ready for maintenance.

Begin Basic Maintenance Program consisting of:

7 a.m.: Take 2 Yeast Away with warm lemon or lime water

8 a.m.: Eat Breakfast of food on the Basic Cleansing Diet (p. 80)—**NO** meat, eggs or dairy). Plus: 1 Willow, 1 Capsicum, 1 Min-Col, 1 Algazim, 1 Rutin, ¼ teaspoon Magnesium Powder

10 a.m.: Drink Cleansing Beverage (as during Intensive) w/juice, clay, psyllium and water.

11 a.m.: Take 2 Pancreatin with lemon or lime water

Noon: Eat Lunch (Basic Cleansing Diet) plus 1 Capsicum, 1 Min-Col, 1 Algazim, 1 Rutin, ¼-teaspoon magnesium powder

2 p.m.: Drink Cleansing Beverage

4 p.m.: Take 2 Pancreatin with lemon or lime water.

5 p.m.: Eat light Supper such as soup and salad

7 p.m.: Take 2 Yeast Away w/warm lemon water 2 hours after eating or taken before bed.

Please practice the following:

- Take a Coffee Enema at least once a daily.
- One hour of quiet time
- One-half hour of walking daily
- Chew food to mush before swallowing
- Drink between meals only

Starting a Second Cleanse

The first cleanse is really a preparation for the second which will produce more results. We encourage a second Seven-Day Intensive Cleanse 7–14 days following the first depending upon individual health requirements.

What happens following a SECOND Seven-Day Intensive Cleanse?

Day 1: Begin **weekly diary** (pp.274-5). By rating how you feel within these categories from 1–10 on the same day of each week, you will be able to track your overall progress. Feel free to add any specific notes for yourself that can be used for further evaluation with a nutritional coach.

Ease back into eating solid food just as advised after the first Seven-Day Cleanse (Appendix G) for **2 days**.

Day 3: Begin Basic Maintenance Program for **3 days**

Day 6: Discontinue Yeast Away and begin the one week Parasite Cleanse (for the first time) in addition to a healthy diet (refer to Changing Our Diet p.158).

Take 1 Willow, 1 Cayenne, 1 Min-Col, 1 Algazim, 1 Rutin and ¼ teaspoon Magnesium once daily after a meal.

Take one Cleansing Drink each day consisting of one-teaspoon of clay, one tablespoon of psyllium in 8–10 oz. green coconut water (if available) or fresh vegetable juice.

The Parasite Cleansing program must be repeated ten days after the first one which means after thirty days you will have completed both the required Parasite Kits.

Between parasite programs resume Yeast Away 1–4 daily plus healthy diet and advised supplements and 1 cleansing drink daily as above. A liver/gallbladder flush as outlined on pages 92-93 might be good for you at this time.

Now you must evaluate your weekly health diary and see if you are improving or declining? This may be the time to do a third Seven-Day Intensive Cleanse or continue to evaluate yourself weekly.

A third cleanse should be done no later than three months after the second and then semi-yearly for health maintenance.

It would also be advisable to begin to keep a record of your urine and saliva pH. I would recommend testing yourself twice weekly, Monday and Thursday, two hours after your mid-day meal. Collect fresh urine in a clean glass jar and saliva on a spoon. Test each by wetting end of a piece of pH test paper strip and compare color on the enclosed chart for numerical reading. A reading of 6.4 for both your urine and saliva would indicate your body is in good balance.

Daily walking is advised. Sweets feed illness. Eat raw almonds and/or raisins by chewing one at a time to mush before swallowing if you crave sweets. Fresh papaya may be eaten after any meal as it aids digestion.

Whenever you drink raw juices—either during or in between cleansing—they must also be consumed properly for the greatest benefit. In a Nutritional Program provided to me by Dr. William Donald Kelley, he states, "They should be sipped slowly to aid the saliva in mixing with the juice. Saliva is still a necessary part of the digestive process and all juices must be thoroughly mixed with saliva before swallowing."

Appendix H: **Personal Weekly Health Progress Record**

DATE	General Well-Being	Energy Level	Aches and Pains	Appetite	Digestion

Rate yourself from 1-10 in each category weekly:

1=Very Poor 5=Fair 10=Excellent

Personal Weekly Health Progress Record Continued

DATE	Bowel Move-ments	Allergies	Weight Changes	Mood Changes	Other

Rate yourself from 1-10 in each category weekly:

1=Very Poor 5=Fair 10=Excellent

Appendix I:

How to Apply Urine Therapy

INTERNAL APPLICATION

Drinking: Morning urine is best. Take the middle stream. You can start with a few drops, building up to one glass a day. Good as a tonic, as a preventative and in minor illnesses.

Fasting: Drink all the urine you pass, except for the evenings, otherwise you won't get any sleep. You can also take some extra water. The urine will quickly change its taste into almost neutral. Fasting on urine and water cleanses the blood. Toxins are removed through liver, skin and out-breath—with exhalation.

Gargle: Beneficial for sore throat, toothache, paradontosis and other ailments of throat, gums and mouth. Urine should be kept in the mouth for 20–30 minutes or as long as possible. Your teeth will stay healthy. After gargling, spit the urine out because it has absorbed toxins and bacteria from the mouth.

Enemas: Urine enemas work very well in cleansing the colon and in providing a direct immune stimulant.

Vaginal douche: Helpful e.g. in yeast problems, white discharge, etc.

Ear and Eye drops: Ear infections; conjunctivitis, glaucoma. For the eyes, dilute the urine with some water.

Sniffing urine or by the use of a “Neti” (a nasal irrigation cup} will relieve sinusitis and other nose problems. It may be diluted with water. It is a very good preventative for colds and air-born allergens and clears the nasal passages.

EXTERNAL APPLICATION

Massaging/Rubbing: You can use either fresh or old urine. Old urine (4–8 days) is generally more effective, but it has a very strong smell. Massaging the whole body is a very important complementary treatment when fasting. It nourishes the body through the skin and helps against increased heartbeat. You can leave the urine on or wash it off after an hour or so, just with water or with a mild, natural soap. Fresh urine as an after shave gives you a beautiful soft skin. But it is also very helpful and healing for all kinds of skin problems: itching, sunburns, eczema, psoriasis, acne, etc.

Gentle rubbing of urine into acupressure points (e.g. on the ears) is very useful when strong allergic reactions take place.

Footbaths: Used for any skin and nail problems of the feet (athletes foot, ringworm, etc.). It eliminates fungus.

Compress: When rubbing is not appropriate, this is another way of applying urine on the skin. Moisten a clean cloth with urine and apply to an area for 15–20 at a time—remoisten as needed. Or, to draw out toxins or poisons from an insect bite for example, you can mix it with a clay powder and apply it like a mask, let dry and leave in place for 15–20 minutes and then wash off.

Hair and Scalp Massage: Renders the hair soft and clean. Sometimes stimulates new hair growth.

Our body produces antibodies as a natural defense against infection and disease. An antigen is a toxic substance or foreign cell that will stimulate the production of an antibody. Studies reveal that urine therapy can aid in the fight against cancer. According to Joseph Eldor, MD at the Theoretical Medicine Institute of Jerusalem, Israel, in his book *Urotherapy for Patients with Cancer,* "Cancer cells release various antigens, some of which appear in the urine. Oral auto-urotherapy is suggested as a new treatment modality for cancer patients. It will provide the intestinal lymphatic system the many tumor antigens against which antibodies may be produced. These antibodies may be transpierced through the blood stream and attack the tumor and its cells."

GUIDELINES AND WARNINGS

It is generally not recommended to combine urine therapy with the use of prescribed chemical, allopathic medicines (conventional western medicine) or recreational drugs. The combination may be dangerous to your health. If you are taking any form of allopathic medicine, begin with the external application (urine massage) until you are free of all medication, if possible. According to reports, there are no side effects from urine therapy, but people may sometimes experience a "healing crisis" (a symptom of illness as the body heals) during the first month.

If it is not possible or safe to stop the use of certain medicines, start with taking a few drops of urine internally or use a homeopathic tincture or gently rub fresh urine into the acupressure points of your ears. Keep looking and feeling very carefully how you and your body are reacting on the treatment. When suffering from a serious illness or, generally, when in doubt, consult a good natural doctor.

Appendix J: **Getting Down to Basics on How to Survive... Who Knows What?**

Much of what is covered in this guidebook depends on the luxury of time and the availability of supplies in order to undo the damage we have done to our bodies and to rebuild our health and immunity to ward off possible chemical and viral attacks while having the strength of body, mind and spirit to stand firm against any opposing force or enemy. What if time is running out? You should be asking, what can be done immediately?

Historically we are offered solutions that treat the symptoms after the fact and rarely are the causes dealt with effectively. Keep in mind that old saying, "an ounce of prevention is worth a pound of cure".

With God by our side, we still need to be physically prepared to do whatever is required to provide the necessities of life for ourselves and our loved ones. Those necessities are good air, water, food, and shelter—in that order.

This book can not possibly be a "be all and end all" on the subject of survival. Thus, we will list some other recommended resources and outline for you what we deem critical to have on hand. We are all probably familiar with the hurricane preparedness supply lists or car emergency kits. I will not go into all of that here. But, I do recommend the following books to acquire:

1. A Bible, Old and New Testament— Through personal study and prayer, develop your relationship with Our Creator, Our Lord and Our Savior.
2. ***A Merck Manual*** (the older the better) or a good nurses or first aide book

3. ***Tom Brown's Field Guide to Wilderness Survival***, Berkley Books, New York, 1983 or ***SAS Survival Guide Handbook***
4. A local medicinal plants reference book
5. ***Build Your Own Earth Oven*** by Kiko Denzer

Recommended tools and supplies:

- Water purifier, such as a "Big Berkey"
- Stored grain and seed—either nitrogen packed, vacuum packed or mixed with diatomaceous earth. This is for sprouting or planting as a survival food. Store canned and dried food as well.
- Multipurpose pocket knife or tool
- Particle or gas mask—in case of contaminated air
- Learn to use a machete and 3-sided file for sharpening it.
- Tent and/or tarps and ropes etc for shelter. Be willing to improvise and utilize natural formations such as caves if accessible. It is always wise to seek higher ground.

Emergency remedies should include:

- Potassium Iodide or Kelp—supplies iodine to protect your thyroid gland against the effects of radiation, and minerals for healthier body function.
- Clay and psyllium—Clay draws out toxins, heavy metals and radiation while the psyllium carries it through and out of the body.
- An enema bag to facilitate detoxification.
- Food Grade Diatomaceous Earth (fossil shell flour) —can be used as a water filter, anti parasite cleanse, healthy food supplement that benefits your body in numerous ways, natural pesticide in the home and garden. Safe for humans and animals—kills

bedbugs, fleas and ticks—taken internally and applied to pets' coats.

- "Oreganol" oil of oregano is a natural antiviral and anti-bacteria remedy for illness and infections.
- Tea Tree oil is a topical antiviral and anti-bacteria remedy.

Most importantly, make an attitude adjustment by giving up your wants, your addictions, and your hang-ups. For instance, your life and the health of your body may someday depend on using your own urine for survival, so be willing to let go of preconceived notions. It is also very likely that survival may depend on the generosity of a neighbor or vice versa—so remember to live by the Golden Rule: treat others as you would have them treat you.

According to Jesus and the ever popular Beatles, "All you need is love, rat-a-tat-ta-ta. All you need is love, love, love is all you need…"

QUESTIONS FOR STUDY

Designed for in-depth discussion in classrooms, study groups or among family members who have read this book

Introduction

1. In what ways did Dr. Keller set himself apart?
2. What significant research by Dr.William Kelley, Dr. Max Gerson and Dr. Bernard Jensen contributed to his plan for wellness?
3. How did God move in his life?
4. What influence did the Amish have on Dr. Keller's outlook?
5. What experiences pertaining to food did he build upon to form his food consciousness today?

Chapter 1: How Our Body Works

1. What evidence is "plain" to us supporting our belief in God's Creation?
2. How does the design of our body affect our health?
3. Name some engineering and scientific principles that occur in the body.

Chapter 2: Why We Get Sick

1. What key factor causes illness and how does it happen?
2. In what areas of our lives do imbalances occur and how are they affected?
3. What modern day advances and medical practices cause us harm?
4. What do we learn from Jesus that can prevent illness?

Chapter 3: How We Can Heal Naturally

1. How does one's faith in God affect one's state of health?
2. How is accepting responsibility for one's health a life-altering experience?
3. Why is the cleansing of the whole body better than treating an ailment?
4. What is the purpose of a nutritionally balanced juicing fast?
5. What contributes to improper digestion and how does this affect our health?
6. Name the organs of detoxification and what role they play.
7. How is administering your own coffee enema beneficial to you?
8. What has supplementation become a substitute for?

Chapter 4: What Is A Healthy Diet?

1. Why was the Garden of Eden an ideal source for food?
2. What problems do local farmers continue to face in today's market?
3. What changes are needed to improve our food supply?
4. Why is eating fresh and raw food better for our health?
5. Why should we avoid processed foods?
6. How does our body's pH balance play a critical role in our health?
7. What food groups are known to be alkaline? Acidic?
8. How does a nursing mother's diet affect her newborn child?
9. What is meant by "food combining"?
10. According to the Bible, is everything God has created good to eat?

Chapter 5: Healthy Food Preparation… Tips from a Chef

1. How does our pattern of eating affect our health?
2. Why is it best to cook vegetables only until tender?
3. What affect does cleansing have on our food cravings?
4. How best should one proportion their meals?
5. How would you approach a change of diet and why?

Chapter 6: How to Eliminate Stress

1. What effect does exercise have on the body?
2. What simple ways can we include exercise into our daily routine?
3. How can we retain our mental capacity?
4. What is a wise investment to make?
5. What are some ways we can downsize and eliminate financial stress?
6. How can we become better neighbors to each other and pool our resources?
7. By partnering with God, how can we be blessed?

Chapter 7: Agriculture, Ecology and You

1. What new concerns arise as we become more in touch with our health?
2. Explain the link between God, the Earth, our food and us.
3. What are the benefits of small family farming?
4. Name four basic requirements for healthful farming.
5. Are we, as Christians, being good caretakers of the land?

Chapter 8: Ideas We Simply Overlook

1. What three important lifestyle modifications would greatly influence our over-all health? How?
2. What three essential needs, critical to our health and survival, were previously discussed?
3. How does dentistry affect our health?
4. What are the advantages and disadvantages to having health insurance?
5. Why is reading and understanding labels important to our health?
6. Would you feel empowered by the use of your own natural medicine?
7. How is the body compared to a storage battery?
8. How is energy being harvested for healing?

Chapter 9: Bringing It All Together

1. Discuss with others the answer to "what is truth?" How is "truth" or "untruth" presented to us today?
2. How are we as individuals just as responsible for the ill effects of the society in which we live?
3. What can we now do to affect change?
4. What do we need to enable us to set ourselves apart?
5. How do the Mennonites set a good example to others?
6. What new commitments are you willing to make for a healthier body and a healthier world?

BIBLIOGRAPHY

The American Heritage Dictionary, 3rd Edition: N.Y. N.Y., Dell Publishing, 1994.

Aihara, Herman. *Acid & Alkaline,* Oroville, CA: George Ohsawa Macrobiotic Foundation, 1980.

Brooks, Linda. *Rebounding to Better Health,* 2nd printing, Albuquerque, NM: KE Publishing, June 1997.

Campbell, T. Colin, PhD. and Thomas M. Campbell II, *The China Study,* Dallas, TX: Benbella Books, 2006.

Cousens, Gabriel, M.D., *Conscious Eating,* Patagonia, AZ: Essene Vision Books, 1992.

Davis, Nord W., Jr., *The Curse Causeless Shall Not Come*, Memorial Edition, Duluth, GA: reprinted by McCoy's Health Center, 1985.

Gerson, Charlotte, and Morton Walker, D.P.M., *The Gerson Therapy,* New York, N.Y.: Kensington Publishing Corp., 2001.

Gerson, Max, *A Cancer Therapy*, 5th Edition, Barrytown, N.Y.: The Gerson Institute in association with Station Hill Press, 1990.

Jensen, Bernard, D.C., with Sylvia Bell, *Tissue Cleansing Through Bowel Management,* 10th Edition: ©Bernard Jensen 1981.

Josephson, Elmer A, *God's Key to Health and Happiness,* Old Tappan, N.J.: Fleming H. Revell Company, 1976.

Kelley, Dr. William Donald, *Nutritional Program* compiled for Dr. Morris Keller, 1969.

The KJV Reference Bible, Grand Rapids, MI: Zondervan, 1994.

Kroon, Coen van der, *The Golden Fountain; The Complete Guide to Urine Therapy,* Mesa, AZ: Wishland Publishing Inc., 2005.

Livingston-Wheeler, Virginia, M.D., and Owen Webster Wheeler M.D., *Food Alive—A Diet for Cancer and Chronic Diseases*, U.S.A.: Livingston-Wheeler Medical Clinic, 1977.

Parham, Vistara, *What's Wrong with Eating Meat?,* 2nd Edition, Corona, NY: PCAP Publications, 1981.

Rand, Howard B., LL.B., *Digest of the Divine Law,* Merrimac, MA: Destiny Publishers, 1943.

Reams, Dr. Carey, with Cliff Dudley, *Choose Life or Death,* Harrison, AR.: New Leaf Press, 1978, © assigned to Holistic Laboratories, 1982.

Shelton, Dr. Herbert M., *Exercise*, Chicago, Illinois: Natural Hygiene Press, Inc., 1971.

Utter, Karen, *7 Vital Laws of Health*, Fort Worth, TX: Natural Solution Training Institute, 1999.

Valentine, Tom, *Microwave Cooking Affects Your Blood*, Search for Health, sample issue.

Walker, Dr. N. W., *The Vegetarian Guide to Diet and Salads*, Phoenix, AZ: O'Sullivan Woodside & Company, 1971.

Wigmore, Ann, *Be Your Own Doctor*, Wayne, N.J.: Avery Publishing Group Inc., 1982.

Wigmore, Ann, *The Wheatgrass Book*, Wayne, N.J.: Avery Publishing Group Inc., 1985.

Index

ABOUT THE AUTHORS

MORRIS F. KELLER is a graduate of Ohio College of Podiatry. A 3rd generation physician/surgeon, he began his own practice in 1963 until diagnosed with cancer in 1969 when he embarked on a new journey of natural healing. Apprenticing under many noted chefs, he became a natural food chef at award winning restaurants in Florida and later in Arkansas where he founded the Mountain View Natural Health Assoc. From 1987–1992 at the Leslie Medical Center in Leslie, Arkansas, he was a consultant in nutrition and researcher in vibrational medicine. He learned the art of baking "Desem" bread in a wood fired oven as a life sustaining food and in 1992 founded Serenity Farm Bread in Leslie, AR. Dr. Keller's ongoing interest in health and nutrition led him to study and cultivate organic agriculture in an Amish community for two years and then partnered with Dharma Farma—organic orchids and gardens in Osage, AR—for eight years. As an active member of the Fayetteville Farmers Market he was elected to the board of directors while also serving as treasurer and President of Arkansas Certified Organic Growers Inc. Today, as Health Missionaries, he and his wife reside in Belize and continue to coach students and give Natural Health Seminars.

KATHRYN ROSE MANDEL-KELLER, wife of Dr. Keller, is a graduate of Queens College, N.Y. with a master's degree in art-education. She has acquired over forty years of experience in diverse sales and marketing along with having used her teaching skills in the N.Y.C. Educational System, in training sales professionals, and in managing a telemarketing department. Her artistry is reflected in her designer, hand knitted hats and handbags once sold at the Fayetteville Farmer's Market, AR. Kathryn has spent the past twelve years learning and putting into practice all that her husband teaches and together they are committed to spreading this knowledge and serving others.

Lightning Source UK Ltd.
Milton Keynes UK
07 February 2011

167064UK00008B/66/P